LYMPHATIC MASSAGE
AFTER PLASTIC SURGERY:

100 MOST COMMON QUESTIONS ANSWERED BY A PLASTIC SURGEON AND A LYMPHATIC MASSAGE THERAPIST

BY MAX YESLEV, MD

BOARD CERTIFIED PLASTIC SURGEON

AND

RUTH MUELLER

LICENSED MASSAGE THERAPIST

ATLANTA, GEORGIA, USA, 2023

FOREWORD:

Our primary intent with this book is to provide readers with cutting-edge knowledge and insights, enabling them to make informed decisions and play an active role in their healing and recovery journey. Additionally, we aim to highlight the potential for achieving optimal recovery outcomes by merging medical interventions with alternative post-operative care. We are dedicated to offering clarity on various topics, including the differences between distinct massage modalities, the nuances of lymphatic drainage therapy, an overview of surgical procedures, aftercare guidelines, self-massage techniques, and general dietary and supplement advice.

We sincerely wish you a successful surgery and swift recovery!

Max Yeslev, MD, Ruth Mueller, LMT

This book is a collection of the most common questions asked by patients who are considering integration of manual lymphatic drainage into their post-surgical recovery routine after cosmetic surgery procedures. Answers to these questions were obtained through detailed research of the most recent medical evidence on MLD techniques, personal observations, direct communication with MLD therapists, and most importantly, from patients' experience. I would like to express my enormous gratitude to Ruth Muller, Jessica Simmons, and Krystle Penn for their dedication, time, and openness in discussing various effects of MLD in postoperative recovery. As a result of their efforts, I constantly continue to learn more about MLD.

I would like to thank my beloved wife, Galina, and daughter, Sophia.

Your unwavering support and patience during the writing of this book have been my anchor. Your love and belief in my vision fueled my motivation and kept me grounded. I am eternally grateful for both of you and feel blessed to have had you by my side throughout this journey.

Max Yeslev, MD

I wish to convey my profound gratitude to Dr. Yeslev for dedicating his invaluable time and effort to addressing queries related to MLD. The driving force behind penning this book has been to enlighten, inform, and provide comprehensive answers to any questions someone might have about healing and recovery pre- and post-surgery. As a skilled plastic surgeon, his expertise is evident. Yet, it's his unwavering commitment to patient care and his generosity in sharing knowledge that truly distinguish him as a pioneer. He champions the integration of traditional medicine with alternative treatments and methodologies.

Dr. Yeslev, please accept my deepest respect and admiration for all that you do.

Blessings to you!

Ruth Mueller, LMT

LEGAL DISCLAIMER:

The content provided in this book on LM after plastic surgery procedures is intended strictly for educational purposes only. It is not meant to diagnose any medical conditions or provide specific treatment recommendations. The information presented in this monograph should not be considered a substitute for professional medical advice, diagnosis, or treatment.

Readers are strongly advised to consult their respective surgeons, certified lymphatic therapists, or qualified healthcare professionals before attempting any techniques or using any products discussed in this book. Every individual's medical condition is unique, and the application of these techniques or products may vary depending on individual circumstances.

The authors and publisher of this book disclaim any liability arising from the use or misuse of the information provided herein. The reader assumes full responsibility for their actions and decisions based on the content of this book.

Readers should always seek professional medical advice and guidance to ensure safe and appropriate care for your specific medical needs. By accessing and using this book, readers acknowledge that they have read and understood this disclaimer, and they agree to adhere to the guidelines set forth herein.

INTRODUCTION

Lymphatic massage (LM), increasingly recognized as an essential component in post-cosmetic surgery recovery, offers significant benefits for various procedures, including liposuction, abdominoplasty and many others. This specialized massage combines manual lymphatic drainage (MLD) techniques with soft tissue manipulation, tailored specifically for postoperative cosmetic surgery patients. However, despite its growing popularity, comprehensive public information on LM remains relatively scarce.

MLD has been historically effective in managing conditions like lymphedema and lipedema. When adapted for post-surgical recovery, this technique was modified to specifically target swelling, making it a widely utilized component of LM in the recuperation process following plastic surgery procedures.

The purpose of this book is to provide an educational resource on the fundamental concepts of this exceptional massage technique. The content of this book is a compilation of answers to the most common questions from patients and clients, which we now wish to share to increase awareness about the benefits of LM in postoperative recovery.

It's important to clarify that "Lymphatic Massage" and "Manual Lymphatic Drainage (MLD)" are distinct terms. While MLD specifically refers to manual massage techniques aimed at enhancing lymphatic flow, postoperative lymphatic massage encompasses a broader range of treatment modalities, including MLD, to facilitate recovery after plastic surgery. To avoid confusion and ensure clarity, we will primarily use the term "Lymphatic Massage" in our discussions and reserve "MLD" for instances where specific details about this technique are necessary to enhance understanding.

It's crucial to clarify that the information in this book is not intended to diagnose, direct readers to self-diagnose, or provide medical advice. Individuals planning cosmetic procedures or recovering from plastic surgery should seek information and guidance from their surgeon or an LM specialist. ALWAYS consult with your healthcare professional to determine if the subjects discussed in this book are applicable to your specific situation.

After reading this book, we hope that those recovering from or planning to undergo cosmetic surgery will gain a better understanding of LM and its potential benefits.

Max Yeslev, MD, Ruth Mueller, LMT

CONTENTS

1

WHAT IS LYMPHATIC MASSAGE AFTER PLASTIC SURGERY?

Lymphatic massage, commonly abbreviated as LM, is a distinct massage therapy method designed to alleviate swelling, whether localized to a specific body part or affecting the body as a whole. The primary goal of an LM therapist is to redirect excessive fluid from the soft tissues into the lymphatic system.

During an LM session, therapists utilize manual lymphatic drainage (MLD) techniques to channel fluid from the target body region into local lymphatic drainage pathways. MLD practitioners employ precise, repetitive strokes on the swollen areas, facilitating the movement of excessive fluid. This fluid is guided through local lymphatic vessels to regional lymph nodes and eventually into the primary lymphatic trunks. Once in the primary trunks, the lymphatic fluid transitions into the systemic bloodstream, where it is ultimately processed and excreted by the kidneys.

MLD massage techniques were initially designed to mitigate the symptoms of lymphedema. This condition is characterized by the excessive accumulation of fluid in specific body regions, often stemming from an impaired lymphatic drainage system due to trauma or surgery. Over time, it became evident that these massage techniques were not only effective for lymphedema but also exceptionally beneficial for postoperative recovery, especially following cosmetic surgical procedures. Implementing MLD techniques after plastic surgery can expedite the resolution of swelling, bruising, and pain. Moreover, MLD massages have the added benefits of reducing inflammation at surgical sites and curbing soft tissue hardening, a condition commonly referred to as fibrosis. Furthermore, post-surgical MLD application can thwart the localized accumulation of fluid in soft tissues, known as seromas. It also refines the appearance of surgical scars and elevates the aesthetic appeal of the treated area.

In the context of postoperative care after plastic surgery, MLD massage techniques—whether used alone or in combination with specialized massage tools—are commonly referred to as "postoperative lymphatic massage" or "postoperative lymphatic drainage massage."

NOTE:

For clarity, within the scope of this book, the term "Lymphatic Massage" (or LM for short) is specifically used to denote either the original or the adapted MLD massage techniques used during recovery after plastic surgery. These techniques, as employed by lymphatic massage therapists—either standalone or in conjunction with massage tools—are aimed at enhancing lymphatic drainage during post-surgical recovery from plastic surgery procedures. Adopting the term LM to collectively refer to the suite of MLD techniques used in postoperative recovery streamlines the content, offering readers a consistent reference and eliminating potential confusion from the sporadic use of varying terms.

Tip:

LM for postoperative recovery significantly differs from conventional massage, which often involves applying forceful pressure to the tissues to achieve deep tissue stretching, especially for muscles. In contrast, LM sessions utilize only minimal to mild pressure applied over the soft tissue, with the primary goal of promoting lymphatic fluid outflow. The objective of LM is the gentle mobilization and transition of excessive body fluid into the lymphatic system and later to the bloodstream. This results in the removal of toxins, metabolic waste material, and excess fluid from the body.

 **LEARN MORE:**

To learn more about the differences between traditional massage and postoperative LM, scan the QR code or click here.

2

HOW IS LYMPHATIC MASSAGE PERFORMED?

During an LM session, the therapist applies gentle pressure and utilizes specific movements to mobilize edema fluid from affected body areas into the lymphatic system. Techniques such as manual gliding, pumping, and tissue stretching are used to assist the transit of fluid into the bloodstream. The specific strokes and techniques applied may vary based on the area of the body being treated and the amount of swelling present.

Typically, the session begins with gentle tapping over the main lymphatic trunk. This is followed by tapping over major lymph nodes located in areas like the neck, armpits, and groin. This process primes the lymphatic system to receive the additional fluid being mobilized from the periphery during the massage. The therapist then performs gentle, light strokes to gradually move excessive body fluid out of swollen areas. This directs the fluid into lymph-collecting vessels and subsequently into regional lymph nodes. After filtration occurs in these nodes, the lymphatic fluid is transitioned into the bloodstream.

Note:

Classic LM techniques, which originated in the 19th century, continue to offer benefits for their original indications, such as non-post-surgical lymphedema. In recent times, many LM therapists have adapted these techniques to more effectively cater to postoperative recovery following plastic surgery. While the specific MLD techniques may differ among providers, the foundational principles of central lymphatic decompression and the gradual fluid mobilization in the soft tissue from proximal to central lymphatic pathways are consistently upheld by LM specialists.

Tip:

When meeting with your LM specialist, it's advisable to request a basic overview of the massage techniques they employ. Ensure that their methods align with the concepts previously described.

LEARN MORE:

Scan the QR code or click here to learn more about LM benefits.

3

WHAT ARE THE BENEFITS OF LYMPHATIC MASSAGE AFTER PLASTIC SURGERY?

LM after plastic surgery offers numerous benefits, such as:

1. Reduces swelling by eliminating excess fluid.

2. Diminishes bruising by clearing blood deposits in tissues.

3. Alleviates pain by reducing edema, bruising, and inflammation.

4. Enhances healing by improving tissue microcirculation and reducing edema.

5. Boosts the immune system by facilitating the influx of immune cells to the surgical area.

6. Decreases inflammation by reducing pro-inflammatory molecules.

7. Stimulates collagen synthesis, aiding in natural recovery mechanisms.

8. Improves skin quality through edema reduction, detoxification, and collagen stimulation.

9. Enhances scar healing by creating optimal conditions.

10. Detoxifies tissues by aiding fluid and debris elimination.

11. Reduces physiological and psychological stress by activating the parasympathetic nervous system.

12. Optimizes body contouring during healing, improving aesthetic results.

13. Reduces soft tissue hardening or fibrosis.

14. Enhances body posture, particularly after abdominoplasty.

Note:

While medical literature does document the benefits of LM, it's essential to recognize that some of the "healing" effects mentioned above are rooted in the personal experiences of massage therapists and their patients. While these firsthand accounts offer invaluable perspectives, they require further scientific evaluation for confirmation. As is the case with all therapeutic methods, continuous research and clinical studies are pivotal in affirming the effectiveness of LM, particularly regarding its impact on post-surgical recovery.

LEARN MORE:

Scan the QR code or click here to learn more about available scientific literature regarding the effects of LM in cosmetic surgery.

4

IS LYMPHATIC MASSAGE NECESSARY AFTER PLASTIC SURGERY?

LM is not mandatory following liposuction or other cosmetic surgical procedures. However, owing to its numerous benefits, LM has become increasingly popular and is often incorporated into postoperative recovery routines. Both plastic surgeons and massage therapists highly advocate for LM as a method to reduce post-surgical edema, thereby enhancing the recovery process. LM is recognized as one of the most potent means to alleviate swelling, accelerate recovery, diminish pain, and achieve superior aesthetic results. However, it's crucial to understand that while LM serves as an effective tool for postoperative recuperation, adhering to standard practices—like wearing postoperative compression garments, maintaining proper nutrition, ensuring adequate water intake, and adjusting physical activity—is equally vital in managing post-surgical swelling.

NOTE:

When administered by a competent professional, LM can be advantageous following nearly all cosmetic procedures. While it's

8

predominantly employed after body surgeries like abdominoplasty (with or without liposuction) and "360 lipo" (with or without buttock fat grafting or BBL), LM also proves beneficial in mitigating edema post-surgery for procedures such as a facelift, arm and thigh lift, breast reduction, mastopexy (breast lift), and many others.

TIP:

Before undergoing any plastic surgery, especially liposuction, engage in a discussion with your surgeon about their stance on postoperative LM. If they advocate for LM, make sure to ask about the ideal locations for the massage sessions and the best time to commence them.

LEARN MORE:

Scan or click here to access a comprehensive list of plastic surgery procedures where LM can aid in recovery.

5

HOW LONG DOES A LYMPHATIC MASSAGE SESSION TYPICALLY LAST?

Typically, one session of LM lasts for one hour, but can vary between 60-90 minutes. The duration may vary depending on individual cases, considering factors such as the body area involved, volume of liposuction, pain levels, and tissue response to the massage. Sessions may be shorter in the early stages of recovery and longer as discomfort improves. For body surgery, most LM specialists recommend at least one full hour-long session to adequately address all affected areas.

Note:

Regular LM sessions aid in reducing inflammation and edema, which are common after surgery. By facilitating the transport of excess fluid and waste into the lymphatic system regularly, LM helps to alleviate swelling and promote a quicker recovery. Additionally, the increased lymphatic flow can enhance the delivery of nutrients and oxygen to tissues, supporting tissue repair and regeneration. Incorporating regular LM sessions as part of the recovery journey can bring about remarkable benefits beyond the reduction of swelling and inflammation. Many individuals experience improved pain relief, enhanced tissue repair, and an overall sense of well-being through the combined effects of LM's gentle yet powerful techniques.

By prioritizing the frequency of LM sessions, one can maximize the potential of this therapeutic modality and foster a harmonious balance within their body's intricate systems. Embracing consistent LM sessions not only aids in postoperative recovery but also paves the way for long-term lymphatic health and improved overall wellness. Everyone's response to LM may vary based on their unique recovery pace and overall health condition. Hence, the guidance of a licensed and experienced LM therapist is crucial in tailoring the treatment plan to suit the specific needs and goals of the client.

Tip:

When discussing LM with your LM therapist, clarify whether the single session appointment time includes only the massage or also accounts for additional time required for entering and leaving the room. After surgery, more time may be spent on preparation and dressing, particularly during the early recovery period. Typically, the LM therapist can assist you with this process, especially when applying compression garments after the massage. Properly preparing for the LM session is essential to ensure a seamless and comfortable experience, and LM therapists are well-equipped to guide and support you through this process. By understanding the timing and procedures involved, you can fully embrace the benefits of LM and focus on your recovery with confidence and peace of mind.

LEARN MORE:

Scan or click <u>here</u> for more information about the typical structure of an LM session.

6

HOW OFTEN SHOULD I GET LYMPHATIC MASSAGE AFTER PLASTIC SURGERY?

Generally, more frequent LM sessions is considered more important to promote recovery than the duration of each individual session. This is because the lymphatic system benefits from consistent and regular stimulation to effectively flush out toxins, excess fluids, and body waste products. Frequent sessions help maintain the momentum of lymphatic fluid flow, enhancing the body's natural detoxification process and promoting a more efficient immune response.

There is no specific number of LM sessions required postoperatively. The recommended number of LM sessions during recovery depends on various factors, such as the type of surgery, volume of liposuction, size of the surgical areas, amount of initial swelling in the surgical area, etc. Frequency of LM sessions is more crucial than duration for achieving better outcomes. In the early postoperative period, LM should be performed more frequently than later in recovery. For example, most LM therapists recommend LM at least three times a week during the first one to two weeks after surgery. As swelling decreases, LM can be performed once a week, and later in recovery once every three to four weeks. Incremental decrease in session frequency varies individually based on the pace of tissue recovery and will be determined by the LM therapist.

Note:

Many plastic surgeons recommend undergoing about ten LMs during postoperative recovery. The suggestion to have "ten postoperative massages" is also frequently mentioned by multiple online sources. However, the origin of this suggestion is unknown, and the rationale behind it remains unclear. While the average number of MLD sessions after surgery typically range from ten to twenty, it is essential to recognize that the exact number of LM sessions recommended during recovery varies significantly based on individual factors and the type of surgery. The optimal number of postoperative massages required should be determined by the MLD therapist during the recovery process, based on the individual progress. Soft issue healing and lymphatic system recovery are slow processes that continue for several months after surgery. Therefore, even after initial visible swelling subsides, intermittent LM sessions later in the recovery process remains beneficial.

Tip:

After a few initial sessions, an experienced LM specialist will gain insights into your tissue's reaction to treatment and can estimate your optimal recovery time. Feel free to ask for a therapist's opinion to help plan your additional treatments and achieve the best results. If you are considering whether to purchase a package of a specific number of massages (for example a ten-massage package deal), it is a good idea to inquire about their policies in case the number of massages needs to be adjusted (either decreased or increased) based on your own recovery progress.

 **LEARN MORE:**

Scan or click here to see recommendations for the frequency of LM sessions after the most common plastic surgical procedures.

7

How much does lymphatic massage cost?

One session of LM can cost, on average, $75-150. The cost may vary based on geographical location, duration, and credentials of the massage therapist. Many LM facilities offer discounted packages of multiple sessions, such as six, eight, ten, or fifteen sessions, providing an opportunity to save on cost. Some plastic surgery offices employ on-site MLD therapists and offer postoperative LM as part of the surgical package. This can have several benefits, including direct contact with the surgical staff and the ability to address healing concerns promptly. Opting for a package deal or LM services at a plastic surgery office can be a wise choice for those seeking convenience and comprehensive support during their recovery journey.

Note:

If you plan to have LM outside of a plastic surgeon's office, it is essential to ensure your comfort during the actual massage session before committing to a large package of LM sessions (such as five, ten, or more). Consider booking a single session initially to evaluate the therapist's approach and your satisfaction prior to booking a costly LM package.

TIP:

Ask about a discount on your first MLD massage. Many LM offices offer discounted rates for the first massage, providing an opportunity to assess whether you are comfortable with the therapist before committing to multiple sessions. Taking this step can help you make an informed decision and ensure a positive experience with your chosen LM specialist.

 **LEARN MORE:** Scan or click here to check the average price for an LM session in each state in the US in 2023.

_8_

WHERE CAN I FIND A QUALIFIED AND EXPERIENCED LYMPHATIC MASSAGE THERAPIST FOR POSTOPERATIVE CARE?

Selecting the right lymphatic drainage therapist is of paramount importance. MLD should only be performed by professionals such as physiotherapists, nurses, occupational therapists, and massage therapists, provided they possess additional qualifications in this area. Ensure that your chosen therapist is not only knowledgeable and experienced in MLD but also routinely works with post-operative patients.

Several national institutions offer certification to therapists upon the successful completion of a specialized forty-hour training in manual lymphatic drainage therapy. These schools place significant emphasis on ensuring therapists' proficiency, understanding of anatomy and physiology, and hands-on training regarding the lymphatic system. Klose Training Program, the Academy of

Lymphatic Studies, and the Norton School are just a few notable examples of such esteemed institutions.

Unfortunately, due to the widespread popularity of post plastic surgery LM treatments, a relatively large number of providers perform LM sessions without the appropriate MLD training and often without basic traditional massage education. Many "body sculpting" businesses include LM as part of their massage services, but lack qualified MLD specialists. Additionally, some of these businesses offer LM "weekend courses" to anyone interested, even without traditional massage training, leading to inappropriately trained and falsely "certified upon graduation" massage providers. While licensed MLD specialists who specialize in LM after cosmetic procedures may charge higher fees, it's not advisable to compromise on the quality of your LM therapist to save on cost. Ensuring your safe recovery and well-being are worth investing in experienced and qualified professionals.

Note:

Many plastic surgeons offer postoperative LM in their practices. LM performed in plastic surgeons' offices is typically carried out by trained professionals who have direct communication with the operating surgeon. Easy access and timely feedback from the treating doctor are significant advantages for both LM and the client. Postoperative LM treatments may also be included in the surgery package as part of the recovery provided by the surgeon's office.

Tip:

Always seek a licensed MLD therapist, regardless of the place they practice. Inquire about the education and training your LM specialist has received, and most importantly, verify if the massage specialist is registered with the state's board of massage therapists. Ensuring their licensure and registration will give you confidence in the expertise and qualifications of the LM therapist.

Finding a qualified and experienced massage therapist can be a daunting task. It's best to ask for a recommendation from your surgeon. It's advisable to explore therapists' websites and read through business reviews. Ensure they have recent and consistent feedback, as this offers insight on the volume of postoperative patients seeking LM among other type of massages.

During your initial communication, inquire if the massage therapist has an electric massage table. Using a motorized electric table allows for comfortable client positioning throughout the session with minimal discomfort. Lastly, review website photos to ascertain the cleanliness and safety standards of the therapist's workspace and facility.

 **LEARN MORE:**

Scan or click here to learn more tips on searching for a qualified MLD specialist for postoperative LM.

2

WHAT ARE THE QUALIFICATIONS OR CERTIFICATIONS TO LOOK FOR IN A LYMPHATIC MASSAGE THERAPIST?

In order to obtain legitimate certification in MLD, an individual must first be a licensed massage therapist or LMT. After completing training in conventional massage techniques, one can pursue further training to obtain MLD certification. When seeking an MLD specialist, it is important to look for a licensed LMT who is also certified in MLD techniques. Being licensed means that the individual has completed standardized courses in MLD and is authorized by the state to practice as a massage therapist. Being certified as an MLD specialist does not automatically guarantee the individual's qualifications or expertise. It is recommended that you inquire about their specific training, experience, and any additional certifications they may hold.

Note:

Some degree abbreviations that can help determine a qualified specialist include:

- CMLDT – Certified Manual Lymph Drainage Therapist
- CMBT – Certified Massage and Bodywork Therapist
- LMT – Licensed Massage Therapist.
- LMBT – Licensed Massage and Bodywork Therapist
- RMT – Registered Massage Therapist
- NCTMB – Nationally Certified in Therapeutic Massage and Bodywork
- BCTMB – Board Certified in Therapeutic Massage and Bodywork.

Tip:

Even if an LM therapist is licensed and well-trained, it is advisable to inquire about the number of postoperative LM sessions they perform on a weekly or monthly basis. The higher the number of LM sessions they perform regularly, the more experienced the therapist is likely to be. This information can provide insight into their level of expertise and familiarity with LM techniques.

LEARN MORE: Scan or click here to find additional information on Board Certified Lymphatic Massage Specialists in your state.

10

HOW SOON AFTER PLASTIC SURGERY CAN I START LYMPHATIC MASSAGE?

The short answer is as soon as your surgeon recommends it. In general, starting LM as early as possible tends to yield better outcomes. Some surgeons recommend starting massage the day after surgery. Ideally, early postoperative massages (within the first three days after surgery) should be performed in the plastic surgery office under the supervision of the doctor. Many LM specialists recommend starting as early as three days after the procedure. Reactive swelling after a surgical procedure typically peaks around day three to four. By minimizing swelling before it reaches its peak, better fluid elimination can be achieved, reducing more prominent postoperative edema. One potential drawback of starting LM early is the possibility of aggravating pain at the surgical sites. However, when performed by experienced LM therapists, even early postoperative massages should not be painful.

Note:

Many plastic surgery offices offer incisional or drain-directed fluid elimination as early as the day after surgery. This technique involves manipulating the surgical area to squeeze out accumulated fluid towards the drain or via an open small incision at the liposuction site, aiding in fluid elimination. An open surgical incision at the liposuction cannula artery point typically naturally closes in twenty-four to forty-eight hours leaving a short opportunity window for fluid elimination. Although such an approach is used by some surgeons, the practice of leaving post liposuction incisions open for the purpose of fluid elimination remains debatable and generally is not advised by most plastic surgeons as leaving the surgical site open after surgery may lead to infection.

TIP:

Before undergoing surgery, consult with your plastic surgeon regarding the timing of your first LM session. If your massage therapist is affiliated with the surgeon's office, consider arranging a call or meeting to delve into the technique and postoperative massage schedule in detail. If you're considering a therapist outside the surgeon's purview, discuss and, ideally, schedule your postoperative MLD sessions as soon as permissible post-surgery. Doing so can ensure you secure your preferred appointment slots.

LEARN MORE: Scan or click here for more tips on preparation for your first LM session.

11

WHAT IS THE RECOMMENDED DURATION FOR LYMPHATIC MASSAGE FOLLOWING SURGICAL PROCEDURES?

The total duration of LM therapy can vary based on several factors. The general principle is to perform more frequent massages shortly after surgery, gradually decreasing frequency as your body recovers, and symptoms such as swelling and bruising improve. Persistent edema or fibrosis may necessitate additional treatment sessions.

Initially, LM is performed up to six times a week, with the frequency decreasing throughout the recovery process. Although individual variation is to be expected, the average frequency of sessions is:

- ▪ - First three weeks: one to three sessions per week
- ▪ - Three to six weeks post-surgery: two sessions every week
- ▪ - Three to six months after surgery: one session every week
- ▪ - Six to twelve months post-op: one session per month as maintenance LM

Note:

During uncomplicated recovery, most people begin to feel like they are "back to normal" approximately three to six weeks after a major plastic surgery procedure. However, the subjective feeling "to be back to normal" does not necessarily indicate completed bodily recovery. In general, soft tissues recover for about a year after surgical trauma. This means that the body can continue to benefit from LM for several months after the initial surgery.

Tip:

Consider scheduling monthly "maintenance" massages for at least the first year after surgery to facilitate your body's full recovery.

 **LEARN MORE:** Scan or click here to learn tips for faster recovery between LM sessions.

12

DOES LYMPHATIC MASSAGE HELP TO REDUCE SWELLING AFTER PLASTIC SURGERY?

Any surgical procedure, regardless of its complexity, invariably alters the body's natural state of balance. One of the most common aftereffects is swelling or edema, which results from an accumulation of fluid in the tissues at surgery sites. In such situations, LM serves as an effective solution by engaging the lymphatic system to address the swelling.

The lymphatic system is a crucial part of our immune system, primarily responsible for carrying waste products and fluids away from the tissues and back into the bloodstream. This system often gets compromised following surgery due to trauma and inflammation, leading to sluggish lymph flow and, consequently, swelling.

During LM the therapist applies gentle, rhythmic pressure on the skin in specific directions to stimulate the flow of lymph fluid. This light pressure targets the superficial lymph vessels just under the skin, effectively moving the stagnant fluid from the swollen area back into the lymphatic system for elimination.

The massage technique generally starts at the site's major lymphatic nodes on the body, such as the neck, armpit, groin and abdominal areas, to "open" the lymphatic system and improve overall lymph flow. The therapist then moves towards the periphery, working on the swollen areas to direct fluid towards these central lymph nodes. This process improves lymphatic circulation, which facilitates the faster removal of waste and inflammatory substances from the tissues, thereby reducing swelling.

Note:

Adding swelling reducing supplements to your daily regimen, in conjunction with LM, can enhance your body's ability to manage swelling even further. Natural supplements known for their anti-inflammatory properties can support the body's healing process, expedite recovery, and help alleviate edema. The most commonly used natural products are Bromelain, Turmeric and Arnica Montana.

Bromelain, found in pineapple stems, helps reduce inflammation and swelling. Turmeric is renowned for its potent anti-inflammatory properties due to the active compound curcumin. Arnica Montana, an herb used in homeopathic medicine, can be taken orally or applied topically to help reduce swelling and bruising. As always, be sure to consult with your healthcare provider before adding any new supplements to your daily routine to ensure they are safe and compatible with your overall recovery plan.

Tip:

Ask your surgeon and LM therapist whether they can recommend postoperative supplements to reduce excessive swelling and follow their recommendations. Remember to drink an adequate amount of water to stay hydrated while taking supplements.

LEARN MORE:

Scan or click here to learn more about supplements to reduce swelling after plastic surgery.

13

CAN LYMPHATIC MASSAGE HELP TO ELIMINATE EXCESSIVE FLUID AFTER PLASTIC SURGERY?

LM plays a significant role in minimizing body fluid retention by facilitating the drainage of excess fluid from tissues. Through gentle and targeted manual techniques, LM stimulates the flow of lymph, a fluid that carries waste products, toxins, and excess fluid away from the tissues. By improving lymphatic circulation, the massage encourages the removal of accumulated fluid, reducing swelling, and promoting a more balanced fluid equilibrium in the body. This process aids in minimizing fluid retention and promoting a healthier, more balanced state within the tissues.

Note:

Hydration plays a crucial role in the effectiveness and safety of LM. During the massage, toxins and waste products are released from the tissues and moved into the circulatory system for elimination. Drinking sufficient amounts of water aids this detoxification process, ensuring these substances are flushed out of the body efficiently. It also helps to prevent dehydration, which could otherwise hinder lymph flow and potentially lead to complications such as fatigue, dizziness, and kidney issues. Therefore, maintaining good hydration after LM not only maximizes the benefits of the therapy but is also crucial for overall health and well-being.

Tip:

Adequate hydration before and after an LM session is extremely important to assist the body in eliminating toxins and removing excess salt, which in turn, facilitates faster healing. Ensure you drink plenty of water before and immediately after the LM session. It's advisable to plan a restroom visit prior to the massage.

LEARN MORE:

Scan or click here to discover the recommended amount of fluids you should drink for optimal recovery post-plastic surgery and during LM sessions.

14

CAN LYMPHATIC MASSAGE HELP WITH PAIN AFTER PLASTIC SURGERY?

LM provides relief from pain after surgery by addressing the underlying causes of discomfort. The gentle and targeted movements used during the massage stimulate the lymphatic system, promoting the removal of excess fluid and reducing tissue swelling. By alleviating swelling and inflammation, LM helps relieve pressure on nerve endings and sensitive tissues, thereby reducing pain. Additionally, the release of endorphins during the massage can further contribute to pain relief and promote a sense of relaxation and well-being. Massage also aids in stretching connective tissue and nerves, enhancing nerve regeneration and maturation, which can lead to a faster reduction in pain during the recovery process.

Finally, soft tissue massage encourages the dilation of blood vessels in the healing tissues. This allows for a more effective delivery of systemic anti-inflammatory medications and supplements through the bloodstream. A more widespread distribution of anti-inflammatory agents in the surgical area results in improved peripheral pain control.

Note:

By targeting areas of postoperative pain and swelling, LM can also improve the overall function of the lymphatic system, enhancing the body's natural ability to heal and repair itself. This can lead to more efficient pain management and a faster recovery overall.

Overall, LM's combination of reducing swelling, stimulating endorphin release, and enhancing tissue recovery makes it a valuable tool in alleviating pain and discomfort after cosmetic surgery. It can significantly improve the postoperative experience and contribute to a smoother and more comfortable recovery.

Tip:

Menthol or CBD-based pain creams and lotions can help alleviate pain and discomfort during recovery after surgery. Applying a pain cream of your choice to the area before an LM session can make the massage experience even more comfortable and minimize any discomfort.

LEARN MORE:

Scan or click here to discover the ten most effective natural pain agents.

15

CAN LYMPHATIC MASSAGE HELP WITH POSTOPERATIVE STIFFNESS AND LIMITED RANGE OF BODY MOTION?

In addition to pain alleviation, LM results in increased flexibility and makes the body feel more comfortable. The physical manipulation of the soft tissues during the massage helps to release muscle tension and increase blood flow to the muscles. This promotes relaxation, reduces muscle stiffness, and enhances overall flexibility. Additionally, massage can improve joint mobility by targeting specific areas of restricted movement and applying techniques that help to release adhesions, and increase the range of motion. The combination of relaxation, improved circulation, and targeted techniques promotes a sense of suppleness and freedom of movement in the body, resulting in increased flexibility.

Note:

There are multiple factors that contribute to decreased body motion, flexibility, and strength following plastic surgery. These factors range from pain at surgical sites to alterations in posture due to surgical procedures such as temporary body bending after abdominoplasty.

In the aftermath of surgery, a patient's resting and sleeping positions may be altered for comfort and safety. For instance, patients may need to sleep with their head elevated or avoid lying on their sides or stomach. This can result in tension and discomfort in muscle groups that are not accustomed to prolonged static positions, potentially causing additional pain.

Extended periods of bed rest and the inability to fully stretch and mobilize muscles due to pain at surgical sites may also contribute to joint stiffness and reduced flexibility. Notably, the body's natural response to injury is to immobilize the affected area to facilitate healing, which can lead to decreased flexibility and range of motion.

A combination of altered body mechanics, prolonged static positions, and the body's natural response to injury can all contribute to the development of stiffness and reduced flexibility after plastic surgery.

Tip:

Consult your surgeon about the exact mobility restrictions during the recovery period and inquire about safe stretching exercises that you can perform postoperatively. Similarly, request guidance from your LM therapist regarding simple stretching exercises that you can do at home to regain your body's pre-operative flexibility level.

LEARN MORE:

Scan or click <u>here</u> to see a stretching guide after body liposuction.

16

CAN LYMPHATIC MASSAGE HELP WITH SKIN IRREGULARITIES AFTER BODY CONTOURING PROCEDURES?

As a result of trauma, the tissue at the liposuction area becomes swollen shortly after the procedure, which may give the impression that the desired results have not been achieved. This swelling can persist for several weeks to up to a year after surgery. Although improvement occurs every day following the procedure, it typically takes three to six months to see the full results. LM, in combination with post-surgical body compression, can significantly expedite the transformation of your body from a swollen state to attractive body curves. Imagine the body areas treated with liposuction like a kitchen sponge soaked with water. By squeezing out all the fluids and allowing the sponge to dry while consistently applying compression, it retains a thin, compact shape. A similar concept applies to the body's recovery after a surgical procedure, particularly liposuction. By eliminating fluid through LM and maintaining proper compression with a garment, treated body areas will assume a more desirable appearance much faster.

Note:

Many experienced LM therapists not only provide massage services but also offer assistance and guidance with postoperative compression garments (also called fajas). They can help adjust the compression garments, focus on providing more compression in specific areas, and provide valuable advice on proper usage.

Tip:

Prior to your surgery, discuss the specifics of post-surgery body compression with your surgeon. Inquire about their recommendations for brands and seek their guidance on sizing. As you recover, you can consult with your LM specialist to assess the degree of compression needed and receive assistance with sizing for the next stage compression garment.

LEARN MORE: Scan or click here to discover more about the benefits of fajas and the different stages of fajas for recovery after plastic surgery.

17

CAN LYMPHATIC MASSAGE HELP TO REDUCE SCAR TISSUE AFTER PLASTIC SURGERY?

LM can be a potent tool in managing and improving the appearance of scars after surgery. Scar tissue forms as part of the body's natural healing process; however, it tends to be less flexible and more fibrous than the original tissue. This can lead to tightness, discomfort, and aesthetic concerns. LM can facilitate the remodeling phase of scar tissue formation, helping to improve its texture, flexibility, and overall appearance.

Specific techniques used in LM, such as counter friction and gentle cupping therapy, help to gently break up fibrosis, the thickening and scarring of connective tissue usually due to injury. This process assists in aligning collagen fibers during the healing process, leading to softer and less noticeable scars. Moreover, LM can stimulate the lymphatic system to carry away waste products around the scar area, reducing inflammation and promoting faster healing. This dual action of enhancing scar tissue remodeling and boosting the body's natural waste disposal system can significantly improve the look and feel of scars post-surgery.

Note:

While LM contributes to less noticeable scarring many LM therapists also include specific scar massages over the surgical scar areas to further improve the appearance of scars. The recovery process for scars is significantly slower and requires concerted effort. Most LM specialists recommend additional at-home scar self-massages to maximize scar reduction after surgery.

Tip:

Ask your surgeon and LM therapist for their recommendations for topical scar reduction products to use for self-scar massages.

 **LEARN MORE:** Scan or click here to discover more about natural anti- scar products for improving the appearance of scars after surgery.

18

WHAT IS CAVITATION AND DO I NEED IT AFTER SURGERY?

Cavitation therapy, often known as ultrasonic cavitation, is a non-invasive cosmetic procedure that uses low-frequency sound waves to break down fat cells under the skin. This process turns the fat cells into free fatty acids, which are easier for the body to flush out through the lymphatic system. Commonly used to eliminate stubborn fat deposits and reduce cellulite, this technique aids in body contouring and skin tightening.

Post-liposuction, cavitation therapy can be particularly valuable. Despite the removal of many fat cells during liposuction, residual fat deposits may remain under the skin, often appearing uneven or lumpy. Cavitation therapy can help smooth out these irregularities, enhancing the overall results of the liposuction procedure. Additionally, it can tighten any loose skin after the procedure, providing a more toned appearance.

However, the decision to use cavitation therapy after liposuction should be made in consultation with your healthcare provider or cosmetic surgeon. Factors such as your overall health, the specific area of liposuction, your body's response to the procedure, and your personal goals for body contouring all play a role in determining if cavitation therapy is suitable for you.

Note:

Although ultrasound cavitation is not a manual lymphatic drainage (MLD) technique, it is often incorporated into postoperative lymphatic massage (LM) sessions. Due to the benefits mentioned above, many LM specialists dedicate time during the massage session to perform ultrasound body cavitation. It's important to understand that cavitation, when used in conjunction with LM, is not performed as a fat reduction procedure but rather as a way to further enhance lymphatic drainage and promote tissue recovery.

Tip:

Ask your LM therapist about additional techniques and equipment, such as a cavitation machine, which can be used during your LM sessions. Inquire also about any additional costs for these services.

LEARN MORE: Scan this QR code or click here to discover more about the benefits of cavitation therapy as part of recovery after plastic surgery.

19

CAN I PERFORM LYMPHATIC MASSAGE ON MYSELF AFTER PLASTIC SURGERY?

Yes, you can perform lymphatic massage (LM) on yourself during recovery after plastic surgery, particularly on your face, neck, upper arms, and abdominal area. Self-LM, or self-manual lymphatic drainage (MLD), can be a beneficial addition to your post-surgery recovery plan. However, it's crucial to first consult with your surgeon or a trained LM therapist. They can instruct you in the correct techniques and movements to ensure you're effectively supporting your lymphatic system without causing harm or discomfort.

Self-LM typically involves gentle, rhythmic movements and stretches on the skin to stimulate lymph flow. It can help reduce swelling, promote healing, and enhance your overall comfort during recovery. However, while it's a valuable complement to professional LM, it shouldn't completely replace treatments provided by a trained specialist. In the early stages of recovery, professional LM treatments can offer more comprehensive support for your healing process. As you progress in your recovery, self-LM can become an increasingly important part of your routine.

Note:

As you further recover from surgery and become more familiar with the techniques used in your LM sessions, you can begin incorporating these techniques more into your at-home self-massage routine.

Tip:

Be proactive. Ask your massage therapist early on to demonstrate a few self-LM techniques that you can perform at home.

 **LEARN MORE:** Scan or click here to discover more about techniques for self-massage.

20

WHAT MASSAGE TOOLS CAN BE USED FOR LYMPHATIC MASSAGE?

During an LM session, therapists often employ a variety of tools to optimize the process and improve results. A commonly used instrument is the LM brush. These brushes, featuring soft and flexible bristles, are crafted to stimulate the lymphatic system gently. Their design ensures they do not cause discomfort or harm to the skin. Typically, therapists use these brushes in soft, circular motions, which aid in promoting lymphatic flow and drainage.

Another popular tool is the massage roller. These can vary from basic handheld rollers to intricate devices with several moving parts. Massage rollers exert consistent, gentle pressure on both the skin and the underlying tissues, facilitating the movement of lymphatic fluid. Furthermore, some LM therapists might incorporate advanced equipment such as ultrasound devices or pneumatic compression devices. These tools are used to further stimulate lymph flow and assist in the elimination of excess fluid. Regardless of the specific tools employed, the primary aim of LM remains consistent: to foster natural lymph drainage, thereby transporting waste products away from the tissues and back into the circulatory system.

Note:

In the period immediately following surgery, LM therapists typically resort only to manual massage techniques. This approach is chosen because manual massage is generally more gentle and causes less discomfort than using massage equipment. As patients recover and their tolerance for pain increases, therapists might begin to integrate additional devices into the treatment based on each patient's needs and objectives. Some of these devices include ultrasound cavitation, cupping, wood therapy, and hot stone treatment.

Tip:

For ongoing care, some LM specialists may recommend specific massagers or tools for home use. It's beneficial to consult with your specialist about which massagers and techniques are suitable for you to use at home, particularly for targeting specific areas.

LEARN MORE: Scan or click here to discover more tools for postoperative LM.

21

WHAT IS CUPPING AND IS IT A PART OF LYMPHATIC MASSAGE?

Cupping therapy is an ancient therapeutic method involving the application of suction to the skin's surface using specialized cups. This suction elevates the skin and underlying tissues, promoting enhanced circulation, muscle relaxation, and relief from tension. Cupping can be performed with stationary or gliding cups.

Cupping therapy can be effectively integrated into lymphatic massage therapy, amplifying its effectiveness in postoperative recovery:

1. **Enhanced Circulation:** Cupping's suction mechanism enhances both blood and lymphatic circulation, facilitating more efficient removal of excess fluid and metabolic waste, especially in areas requiring lymphatic drainage.

2. **Tension Release:** Cupping contributes to the relaxation of muscles and fascia, which may become tense and restricted after surgery. This relaxation aids in reducing discomfort and promoting overall well-being.

3. **Improved Lymphatic Drainage:** The suction action of cupping stimulates lymphatic vessels, encouraging the movement of lymphatic fluid. This is particularly beneficial in reducing postoperative swelling and edema.

Benefits of Cupping in Postoperative LM include:

1. **Edema Reduction:** Postoperative swelling is a common concern. Cupping enhances lymphatic flow, expediting the reduction of swelling and promoting a speedier recovery.

2. **Pain Management:** Cupping can alleviate postoperative discomfort and pain by relaxing tense muscles and increasing local blood flow.

3. **Accelerated Healing:** The combined approach of lymphatic massage and cupping supports a faster healing process, allowing patients to resume normal activities more quickly.

4. **Scar Management:** Cupping can be applied around surgical incisions to promote scar tissue healing. Improved circulation facilitates the delivery of essential nutrients to the scar tissue, aiding in the healing process.

Note:

Cupping therapy, when integrated into lymphatic massage, offers a valuable means of optimizing postoperative recovery following plastic surgery. Its ability to enhance circulation, alleviate swelling, manage pain, and support the healing process makes it a compelling choice for individuals seeking expedited recovery and optimal surgical outcomes. Choosing a skilled therapist with experience in both cupping and LM ensures a safe and effective treatment plan tailored to the patient's unique requirements.

Tip:

Cupping should be employed with caution, typically in the later stages of postoperative recovery. An experienced therapist is essential to carefully control the degree of cup suction, particularly during the initial phases after surgery when the surgical site is more sensitive. However, it is a valuable tool for preventing and treating issues such as fibrosis, scarring, and surface irregularities of the skin when used in conjunction with LM.

 **LEARN MORE:** Scan or click here to learn more about benefits of cupping in postoperative recovery.

22

CAN LYMPHATIC MASSAGE HELP WITH THE RESOLUTION OF POSTOPERATIVE FIBROSIS OR ADHESIONS?

LM, when combined with light deep tissue techniques, plays a pivotal role in managing fibrosis after liposuction. The systematic, rhythmic strokes of LM are effective in breaking down fibrous tissues, thus enabling the body to naturally eliminate these harder, denser areas. By boosting lymphatic circulation, LM not only supports the body's inherent healing processes but also assists in softening fibrotic tissue, thereby improving skin texture.

Furthermore, LM enhances circulation to the affected areas, ensuring better blood flow. This increased circulation brings more nutrients and oxygen to the healing tissues, fostering cellular health and recovery. In fibrotic areas, this enhanced circulation can stimulate collagen and elastin production—proteins crucial for maintaining skin elasticity and resilience. Consequently, LM, in conjunction with firmer and deeper massage strokes, can significantly alleviate the effects of fibrosis, rendering the skin smoother and more supple.

LM is also beneficial in reducing inflammation, often a precursor to fibrosis. By facilitating the removal of waste products and excess fluid, the massage helps minimize inflammation, which in turn can reduce the likelihood of fibrosis development. However, it's important to recognize that while LM is highly advantageous, it is not a standalone solution. The most effective results from LM are observed when it is part of a comprehensive post-operative care regimen, which may include wearing compression garments, maintaining a balanced diet, and staying hydrated. Regular consultations with healthcare providers are essential to monitor progress and adjust care plans as needed.

Note:

The primary objective of early LM is the prevention of fibrosis. Despite comprehensive LM, fibrosis can still develop during recovery. It's crucial to incorporate early detection and implement specific techniques targeting fibrosis reduction in postoperative LM care. Fibrosis is a persistent issue that resolves gradually and demands concerted effort from both the patient and the LM therapist. The presence of fibrosis, despite LM treatments, is not indicative of LM ineffectiveness. Persistence and regular application of massage techniques typically lead to a favorable outcome.

Tip:

While your LM therapist will assess your body for fibrotic areas, you are the one who is most familiar with your own body. If you notice knots or tender lumps at the liposuction sites, inform your specialist promptly. Early identification and treatment of these areas can make a significant difference.

 **LEARN MORE:** Scan or click <u>here</u> to learn how to do self-exams to help diagnosis of fibrosis areas.

23

CAN LYMPHATIC MASSAGE HELP WITH BRUISING AFTER PLASTIC SURGERY?

Yes, LM can indeed aid in resolving bruises following plastic surgery. Bruising results from trauma to blood vessels during the surgery, causing blood to leak into adjacent tissues. LM assists in reducing bruising through several mechanisms:

1. **Improved Lymphatic Flow:** LM stimulates the lymphatic system, vital for clearing cellular waste and excess fluids, including leaked blood during surgery. Enhanced lymphatic flow through LM helps to more efficiently remove accumulated blood from bruised areas.

2. **Enhanced Circulation:** LM also boosts circulation, aiding in the clearance of stagnant blood. Improved blood flow delivers fresh oxygen and nutrients to the tissues, speeding up healing and diminishing the appearance of bruises.

3. **Reduced Inflammation:** By clearing inflammatory substances and promoting natural healing processes, LM helps reduce inflammation in bruised regions.

4. **Gentle Stimulation:** The gentle nature of LM ensures that bruised tissues are not further aggravated. The light, rhythmic strokes promote the body's natural drainage mechanisms without additional harm.

5. **Early Intervention:** Implementing LM shortly after surgery can prevent severe bruising by facilitating efficient blood removal from tissues before significant discoloration occurs.

Note:

Another often overlooked advantage of LM during post-surgery recovery is the alleviation of postoperative pain. Enhancing lymphatic flow and stimulating blood circulation via LM reduces swelling, subsequently diminishing pain at surgical sites. Moreover, LM aids in relieving muscle tension and triggers endorphin release, which can significantly lessen postoperative pain. Thus, LM might contribute to a decreased dependence on narcotic-based pain medications.

Tip:

Monitor your pain medication regimen closely and discuss the possibility of transitioning to non-narcotic pain relief as soon as feasible with your healthcare provider. If pain medications are recommended by your surgeon, it's wise to obtain them before your surgery to ensure availability when needed. Additionally, consider requesting prescriptions for a muscle relaxer and a stool softener as preventive measures for potential post-operative needs.

 **LEARN MORE:** Scan or click <u>here</u> to find out more about benefits of LM for pain reduction after surgery.

24

HOW DOES LYMPHATIC MASSAGE HELP WITH POSTOPERATIVE RECOVERY?

LM plays a crucial role in postoperative recovery after plastic surgery by promoting a faster and smoother healing process. Here are the key ways in which LM helps:

1. **Reduces Swelling:** Postoperative swelling, also known as edema, is a common concern after plastic surgery. LM uses gentle, rhythmic strokes to stimulate the lymphatic system, encouraging the removal of excess fluid and waste products from the surgical area. This leads to a significant reduction in swelling and discomfort.

2. **Enhances Lymphatic Drainage:** The lymphatic system is responsible for maintaining fluid balance in the body and supporting the immune system. LM aids in improving lymphatic drainage, enabling the body to clear away toxins and cellular debris more efficiently.

3. **Speeds up Healing:** By facilitating the removal of waste and excess fluid, LM accelerates the body's natural healing process. This means that tissues are repaired faster, leading to quicker recovery and reduced downtime after surgery.

4. **Minimizes Scar Tissue Formation:** Gentle manipulation of the tissues during LM can help prevent the formation of excessive scar tissue. This promotes a smoother and more aesthetically pleasing healing of the surgical incisions.

5. **Improves Circulation:** LM enhances blood circulation in the treated area, increasing oxygen and nutrient supply to the healing tissues. Improved circulation also helps to flush away inflammation, further aiding in the healing process.

6. **Eases Pain and Discomfort:** By reducing swelling and improving circulation, LM can alleviate postoperative pain and discomfort. This provides patients with greater comfort during the recovery period.

7. **Supports Immune Function:** A properly functioning lymphatic system is vital for a robust immune response. LM boosts the immune system, helping the body ward off infections and heal more effectively.

8. **Promotes Relaxation and Well-Being:** The gentle, soothing nature of LM promotes relaxation and reduces stress, which can be beneficial for both physical and emotional well-being during the recovery process.

9. **Personalized Treatment:** LM is tailored to each patient's specific needs and the type of surgery they underwent. This personalized approach ensures that the massage is safe, effective, and appropriate for the individual's condition.

NOTE:

The term "recovery after surgery" refers to the period following a surgical procedure during which the body heals and returns to a state of normal functioning. It encompasses the time it takes for the surgical site to heal, for any incisions to close, and for the body to regain strength and function. The time and process for recovery after surgery can vary widely depending on the type of surgery performed, the individual's overall health and condition, and the complexity of the procedure.

During the recovery period, the body goes through various stages of healing, which may include reducing swelling and inflammation, repairing tissues, regaining mobility, regaining normal body posture and function, and managing any pain or discomfort. The length of the recovery period can range from days to weeks or even months, depending on the extent of the surgery and the body's individual response to the procedure.

Proper postoperative care, including following the surgeon's instructions, taking prescribed medications, attending follow-up appointments, and engaging in recommended rehabilitation or therapy, all play crucial roles in the recovery process. The goal of recovery after surgery is to ensure the best possible outcome, minimize complications, and allow the individual to resume their normal activities and quality of life as soon as possible.

TIPS:

One way to evaluate the effects of LM on individual recovery is to read through reviews of massage offices specializing in postoperative LM. These reviews can provide valuable insights into the experiences of others who have undergone similar procedures and received LM as part of their recovery process. Additionally, social media platforms offer a wealth of information and personal accounts of individuals who have undergone plastic surgery and utilized LM as part of their postoperative care. Joining social media support groups dedicated to recovery after plastic surgery or specific procedures can be particularly helpful in obtaining more in-depth information and firsthand experiences from others who have benefited from LM.

In these online communities, individuals often share their recovery journeys, including how LM has played a role in their healing process. You can learn about the various benefits and potential challenges of LM from people who have already undergone the procedure you are considering. By interacting with others in these communities, you can ask questions, seek advice, and gain a deeper understanding of how LM may impact your own recovery.

 **LEARN MORE:** Scan or click here to learn more about benefits of LM in recovery after plastic surgery.

25

ARE THERE ANY POTENTIAL RISKS OR ADVERSE EFFECTS LINKED TO UNDERGOING LYMPHATIC MASSAGE FOLLOWING PLASTIC SURGERY?

LM, when performed by a certified and trained professional, is generally considered safe and beneficial for post-operative recovery. However, like any therapeutic intervention, it is not entirely without risks or potential side effects.

In some cases, individuals may experience temporary side effects such as light-headedness or fatigue immediately after the massage session. This can be attributed to the release of stored toxins and waste products from the tissues into the bloodstream, which are then eliminated by the body's detoxification processes. Ensuring proper hydration before and after the session can help to mitigate these effects.

Another potential risk includes exacerbation of pre-existing conditions. For instance, patients with heart or kidney conditions, or those with deep vein thrombosis, may not be suitable candidates for LM as this therapy can potentially overload their already compromised systems. In such cases, the treatment should only be performed under the supervision of a healthcare professional. Furthermore, it is crucial to avoid applying pressure to surgical incisions or areas of active inflammation or infection to prevent exacerbating these conditions. As with any post-operative care, it's essential to communicate openly with your healthcare provider about your health history and current conditions to ensure that LM is a safe and effective part of your recovery process.

Note:

In the presence of chronic health or medical problems prior to surgery, it is essential not only to discuss them with your surgeon and LM therapist but also with your personal medical doctor. Certain medical conditions may require special considerations when it comes to receiving LM after surgery, as they can potentially impact the treatment or result in complications. Your medical doctor can provide valuable insights and guidance to help determine if LM is suitable for you and if any modifications or precautions need to be taken to ensure your safety and well-being during the postoperative period.

Tip:

If you have multiple medical problems, feel free to discuss whether LM is suitable for you with your primary care doctor. You can even facilitate a direct discussion between your doctor and LM therapist to explore whether LM can be beneficial for you. Open communication between your healthcare providers can help ensure that all aspects of your medical history and needs are considered when incorporating LM into your healthcare plan.

 **LEARN MORE:** Scan or click here to learn about specific side effects of LM.

26

ARE THERE SPECIFIC RECOMMENDATIONS OR PROTOCOLS TO FOLLOW BEFORE OR AFTER RECEIVING A LYMPHATIC MASSAGE SESSION?

Before Your LM Session:

1. **Stay Hydrated:** Drink ample water prior to your session. Hydration assists in lymphatic drainage, aiding your body's circulation and waste elimination processes.

2. **Comfortable Clothing:** Choose loose, comfortable attire for your appointment, facilitating ease of movement.

3. **Avoid Heavy Meals:** Opt for a light snack over a heavy meal before your massage to prevent discomfort.

4. **Inform Your Therapist:** Share your medical history, current health status, and any areas of discomfort or pain.

This information enables your therapist to tailor the session for optimal benefit.

5. **Address Any Concerns:** It's natural to feel anxious or sore, especially if you're recovering from surgery. Your therapist is experienced with postoperative care and will ensure your comfort on the massage table. Expect to lie on an electric massage table that allows for various positions. For example, post-BBL (Brazilian Butt Lift) patients may be massaged while standing, kneeling, or sitting with a BBL pillow under the hamstrings to protect the grafted fat cells.

6. **Preparation for the Session:** The therapist will guide you to undress (typically to your underwear) and lie on the massage table, your body will be covered with a sheet or draping. The electric table can be adjusted for your comfort, especially if sitting normally is uncomfortable post-surgery.

During Your LM Session:

1. Making sure you choose an LM therapist with experience working with clients recovering from the same type of surgery you've had will ensure they tailor your treatment based on your needs and you will be comfortable throughout the process. Feel free to express preferences regarding table temperature, massage pressure, positioning, oils, and aromatherapy use.

2. Discuss your pain level, discomfort areas, and recovery experience. Open communication with your therapist helps them adjust their techniques to increase the benefits from each session.

3. Should you feel any discomfort, immediately inform your therapist. LM is a gentle technique and should not cause pain.

The therapist may adjust pressure or technique according to your feedback.

After Your LM Session:

1. **Continue Hydrating:** Drink water post-session to help eliminate toxins released during the massage.

2. **Rest:** Allow time for rest if you feel tired after the massage.

3. **Monitor Your Body:** Observe any unusual reactions post-massage and inform your therapist or doctor as needed.

4. **Regular Sessions:** Follow your therapist's advice on the frequency of sessions for the best results.

5. **Healthy Diet:** Consume a balanced diet to aid recovery and lymphatic function. Avoid processed foods, excessive sodium, and alcohol.

Note:

These are general suggestions. Always adhere to the specific advice of your healthcare provider or LM specialist. Your LM therapist will provide the most effective guidelines tailored to your situation.

Tip:

Review and incorporate the guidelines provided by your LM office into your surgeon's postoperative instructions. Consult your healthcare professionals for any concerns or clarification to ensure a smooth recovery.

LEARN MORE: Scan or click here to view a checklist to help you prepare for your first LM session.

27

ARE THERE ANY CONTRAINDICATIONS OR PRECAUTIONS FOR LYMPHATIC MASSAGE AFTER PLASTIC SURGERY?

LM is a generally safe and beneficial procedure for most individuals recovering from plastic surgery. However, there are certain contraindications and precautions that patients and therapists alike should be aware of to ensure optimal results and avoid potential harm.

Firstly, it's important to note that LM should not be performed on areas of the body where there is an infection, acute inflammation, thrombosis or a malignant disease. These conditions can potentially be exacerbated by LM, as the procedure might facilitate the spread of the harmful agents, thereby complicating the patient's health status. Also, LM should not be performed too soon after surgery as it can potentially interfere with the healing process. It is crucial to receive approval from the surgeon before beginning any massage treatments.

Note:

Patients should always inform their therapist about any pre-existing health conditions, such as heart disease, kidney disease, or other serious conditions. Individuals with these conditions may need to avoid or modify certain treatments as they could potentially overtax the circulatory system or interfere with medication regimens. While LM is a gentle technique, any form of bodywork can have systemic effects, and these need to be factored into the overall treatment plan. Therefore, open communication between surgeon and therapist is essential to ensure safe and effective treatment.

Tip:

You should always obtain permission to start LM not only from your plastic surgeon but also from your primary care doctor if you have an underlying or chronic medical condition.

LEARN MORE: Scan or click here to find out more about conditions where LM is contraindicated.

28

How soon can I expect to see results from lymphatic massage after plastic surgery?

LM is a therapeutic process, and, like most therapies, the results are not typically instantaneous but are seen gradually over time. The timeframe in which individuals notice improvements varies, largely depending on the extent of the surgery, the individual's overall health, and the consistency of the massage sessions.

Immediately following an LM session, patients often report feeling a sense of lightness or relief in the massaged area, as well as a general sense of relaxation. However, when it comes to measurable improvements such as decreased swelling, increased mobility, or reduced pain, it generally takes a series of consistent sessions to observe notable changes. It's not uncommon to see gradual improvement after each session, with significant changes being more apparent after a few weeks of regular LM treatments.

That said, every individual's body responds differently to both the surgery and the recovery process. Factors such as the patient's overall health, age, lifestyle habits (like diet and exercise), the type of surgery undergone, and adherence to post-operative instructions can all play a significant role in recovery time and the effectiveness of LM. It's essential to keep in mind that LM is a supportive therapy designed to aid and accelerate your body's natural healing process, and patience is often key to seeing optimal results.

Note:

It can be challenging for patients to notice improvements in bruising, swelling, and body shape, as they see their bodies every day. The recovery process is gradual and may not be noticeable on a day-to-day basis.

Tip:

Take the initiative to ask your LM therapist to take pictures after each LM session or every week. This will allow you to easily track your body's progress in terms of decreased bruising and swelling during the recovery period, especially when compared to the first picture taken at the very beginning of your recovery journey.

LEARN MORE: Scan or click here to find out if LM is working for you.

_29_

IS LYMPHATIC MASSAGE COVERED BY INSURANCE AFTER PLASTIC SURGERY?

In many instances, LM after plastic surgery is viewed as a non-medical, elective treatment, and therefore, most insurance companies do not cover this service. Insurance coverage typically focuses on procedures and treatments deemed medically necessary, and while LM can certainly aid in the recovery process after plastic surgery, it is often classified as a wellness or self-care treatment. Thus, out-of-pocket payment is often required.

However, there can be exceptions depending on your individual insurance plan and the reasons for your surgery. For instance, if the surgery was reconstructive in nature, or performed to improve function or alleviate health issues (as opposed to being purely cosmetic), your insurance might cover LM as part of your rehabilitation program. It's important to note that each insurance policy differs significantly, so what applies to one may not apply to another.

It is strongly recommended that you speak directly with your insurance provider to determine the specifics of your coverage. You may also need a letter or prescription from your doctor or surgeon outlining the medical necessity of the LM for your recovery. Remember, every insurance plan is unique, so even if LM isn't typically covered, there may be avenues to explore to secure partial or full coverage for your post-surgical treatment.

Note:

LM treatments can sometimes be paid for through a Flexible Spending Account (FSA), Health Savings Account (HSA), or Health Reimbursement Account (HRA). These are special accounts that individuals can contribute to, tax-free, for use on certain out-of-pocket health care costs.

However, the specific eligibility of LM for coverage under these plans can vary based on individual circumstances and the rules of your specific account. It's often necessary to have a Letter of Medical Necessity (LMN) from your healthcare provider stating that the LM is a necessary part of your post-operative recovery.

Tip:

Always consult with your plan administrator or the provider of your FSA, HSA, or HRA to understand what expenses are covered and what documentation you might need to provide. It's also beneficial to consult with your tax advisor to understand any potential tax implications.

LEARN MORE: Scan or click here to find out how LM can be approved by medical insurance.

30

WHAT IS THE DIFFERENCE BETWEEN LYMPHATIC MASSAGE AND REGULAR MASSAGE TECHNIQUES?

LM and regular massage, such as Swedish or deep tissue massage, have different goals and employ distinctive techniques, although they may seem similar to the untrained eye.

LM using MLD techniques is a specialized form of massage that aims to stimulate the lymphatic system, promoting the flow of lymph fluid. This is crucial for the body's defense system as it helps to remove waste, toxins, and excess fluids from the body's tissues. MLD is gentle, rhythmical, and has a soothing, calming effect on the nervous system. It targets the superficial lymphatic network located just under the skin. The main goal of MLD is to reroute the lymph flow around blocked areas into healthy lymph vessels, thus facilitating the drainage of stagnant and toxic fluid.

On the other hand, traditional massage techniques, such as Swedish or deep tissue massage, primarily focus on relieving tension in the muscles, promoting relaxation, and enhancing overall well-being. These techniques tend to use deeper pressure and include a variety of strokes such as kneading, friction, compression and stretching to address issues in the musculoskeletal system.

While both MLD and regular massage can promote relaxation and wellness, they each have distinct benefits and uses. Traditional massage is excellent for reducing muscle tension and stress, while MLD is particularly beneficial for conditions involving swelling, fluid retention, and certain types of surgery recovery, including plastic surgery.

Note:

A massage therapist certified in LM and a regular massage therapist have different areas of expertise and require distinctive training and certification paths, highlighting the importance of selecting a specialist suitable for your needs.

A regular massage therapist typically specializes in various techniques designed to help reduce muscle tension, stress, and promote overall wellness. Their training focuses on understanding the human musculoskeletal system, identifying tension points, and learning techniques to alleviate discomfort or pain. Regular massage therapists may specialize in numerous types of massages such as Swedish, deep tissue, sports massage, and more. Certification for regular massage therapists involves a standard course and examination that varies depending on the regulations of the specific country or state.

On the other hand, an LM therapist specializes in stimulating the lymphatic system to aid the body in removing toxins, waste, and excess fluids. To become a certified MLD therapist, one must undergo additional, specialized training that includes studying the lymphatic system in-depth, learning specific techniques to stimulate lymph flow, and understanding how to address various health conditions related to lymphedema or post-operative recovery. After this training, therapists must pass an examination to demonstrate their knowledge and skills in MLD.

The specific training and certification required for MLD therapists underscore the complexity of the lymphatic system and the precision required in performing LM.

Tip:

When choosing a therapist for lymphatic drainage post-surgery, it's crucial to ensure that they have the proper certification and experience in MLD. This will provide the assurance that they have the specialized knowledge and techniques necessary to help optimize your recovery process.

 **LEARN MORE:** Scan or click here to find out when regular deep tissue massage can be safely done after a tummy tuck.

31

CAN LYMPHATIC MASSAGE HELP WITH POSTOPERATIVE INFLAMMATION?

Yes, LM can indeed help with postoperative inflammation. Following surgery, the body naturally responds to inflammation and swelling, which are part of the healing process. However, excessive swelling can lead to discomfort and slow down recovery.

LM works by stimulating the lymphatic system, which is responsible for removing waste products and excess fluids from body tissues. By facilitating the efficient flow of lymphatic fluid, these massages can help to reduce the accumulation of fluid in the tissues, thereby lowering inflammation.

Furthermore, LMs are often gentle, using light, rhythmic strokes that help to encourage the drainage of lymph without causing additional trauma to the surgical site. This gentle approach is particularly beneficial in the postoperative setting, as it aids in reducing inflammation without causing further discomfort or disruption to the healing process.

Note:

While LM can play a critical role in managing postoperative inflammation, it should be part of a broader post-surgical care plan. Adequate rest, good nutrition, staying hydrated, and following all your healthcare provider's instructions are all crucial for an optimal recovery. Always consult with your healthcare provider or a trained MLD therapist before starting LM after surgery.

Tip:

Some additional measures to reduce postoperative inflammation include:

1. **Proper Hydration:** Staying hydrated is crucial for supporting your body's natural healing processes, including the reduction of inflammation. Drinking enough water can help flush toxins and excess fluids out of your body, reducing swelling and inflammation.

2. **Diet:** Certain foods are known to have anti-inflammatory properties. Incorporating them into your diet can help reduce post-surgery inflammation. These include fruits such as blueberries and oranges, vegetables like spinach and broccoli, fatty fish, nuts, and olive oil. On the contrary, try to avoid foods that can increase inflammation, like fried foods, sugar-sweetened beverages, and processed foods.

3. **Rest and Elevation:** Giving your body the proper time to heal and recover is important in reducing inflammation. Additionally, depending on your surgical procedure, elevating the surgery area can help to reduce swelling by promoting the drainage of excess fluids.

4. **Gentle Exercise:** Once cleared by your doctor, gentle movement and exercises can help reduce inflammation. This

doesn't mean strenuous activity, but rather light movements such as walking or doing approved gentle stretches, which can improve blood circulation and reduce swelling.

5. **Supplements:** Certain supplements are known to have anti-inflammatory properties. However, always check with your healthcare provider before starting any new supplement regimen. Some commonly used supplements include:

   o Bromelain: This enzyme found in pineapples is often used to reduce inflammation and swelling.

   o Turmeric (Curcumin): The active compound in turmeric, curcumin, has strong anti-inflammatory effects.

   o Omega-3 Fatty Acids: Found in fish oil, these have anti-inflammatory properties and are widely used to manage inflammation.

   o Quercetin: A plant pigment found in many plants and foods, quercetin possesses antioxidant and anti-inflammatory effects.

   o Vitamin C: Besides its role in boosting the immune system, vitamin C can also help to reduce inflammation.

Remember, it is essential to check with your healthcare provider before starting any new dietary regimen or supplement intake, especially after surgery. They can provide personalized advice based on your health condition and surgical procedure.

 **LEARN MORE:** Scan or click <u>here</u> to learn about more ways to decrease body inflammation after plastic surgery.

32

HOW DOES LYMPHATIC MASSAGE PROMOTE DETOXIFICATION AFTER SURGERY?

LM promotes detoxification after surgery by stimulating the lymphatic system, an essential part of the body's immune system. The lymphatic system helps in the removal of waste products, toxins, and excess fluids from the body's tissues. It consists of a network of vessels and nodes that carry a clear fluid called lymph, which contains white blood cells to fight infection and proteins and fats to supply nutrients.

During an LM, a trained therapist uses a series of gentle, rhythmic movements to stimulate the flow of lymph. This manual stimulation aids the lymphatic system to efficiently drain away the waste products and toxins from the tissues, essentially assisting with the body's natural detoxification process. After surgery, there can be an accumulation of metabolic waste products in the tissues due to inflammation and the body's healing process. By encouraging lymph flow, LM can help to expedite the removal of these waste products.

Furthermore, by reducing the buildup of waste products, LM can help to decrease inflammation and swelling, common side effects of surgery. This reduction in inflammation further supports the detoxification process as it allows for improved circulation and oxygenation of the tissues, facilitating more efficient removal of waste products. Consequently, the detoxification promoted by LM can contribute to a faster recovery process after surgery and enhance overall well-being.

Note:

Some additional ways to enhance body detox while recovering after plastic surgery include:

1. Hydration: One of the most straightforward ways to enhance detoxification after surgery is to maintain proper hydration. Water helps to flush out toxins and waste from the body and promotes optimal functioning of the kidneys, organs essential in the body's detoxification process. Aim to drink enough water each day, bearing in mind that individual needs may vary.

2. Balanced Diet: Consuming a diet rich in fruits, vegetables, lean proteins, and whole grains can provide your body with the necessary nutrients for detoxification. These foods contain antioxidants and fiber, which aid in the elimination of toxins. Incorporating foods high in vitamin C, such as citrus fruits, can also support the body's natural detox mechanisms.

3. Exercise: As your body recovers and with your doctor's approval, gentle exercise can help stimulate the lymphatic system, much like LM does. Activities such as walking or gentle yoga can encourage circulation and lymph flow, assisting in the removal of toxins.

4. Deep Breathing and Relaxation Techniques: Deep breathing or meditation can help reduce stress levels. Stress can hinder the body's detoxification processes, so promoting relaxation can indirectly support detoxification.

5. Supplements: Certain supplements can aid in the body's detoxification process. For example, milk thistle is known for its liver-supporting properties, as it can help to detoxify and reduce inflammation in the liver. Similarly, turmeric has potent anti-inflammatory and antioxidant effects that can support detoxification. However, always consult with your doctor before starting any new supplement regimen, especially during the recovery period after surgery.

Tip:

Ask your doctor and LM therapist whether certain detox products such as detox tea, smoothies, or green powders can be helpful in your recovery.

LEARN MORE: Scan or click here to learn more about top natural detox herbal supplements.

33

ARE THERE ANY PRECAUTIONS TO TAKE DURING LYMPHATIC MASSAGE IF I HAVE EXISTING MEDICAL CONDITIONS?

Yes, there are several precautions to consider when undergoing LM after plastic surgery if you have existing medical conditions. The lymphatic system is complex and plays a vital role in your overall health, so it's crucial to communicate any existing conditions to your therapist.

Firstly, patients with heart disease or circulatory problems need to take special precautions as manipulating the flow of fluid in the body can put additional strain on the heart. In such cases, the therapist should adjust the intensity and technique to accommodate the condition.

Secondly, those with infections, especially those that are not being treated, should avoid LM as it could potentially spread the infection throughout the body. The same applies to individuals with a fever or acute inflammation, as these may be signs of an ongoing infection.

Lastly, patients with a history of blood clots or deep vein thrombosis should be aware that LM can, in rare cases, potentially dislodge a clot which could lead to serious complications such as a pulmonary embolism.

Note:

In all cases, it's essential to consult with your healthcare provider before starting LM therapy. They can provide personalized advice based on your medical history and current health status. Regular communication with your massage therapist is also crucial as this will allow them to adapt their techniques to best suit your needs and ensure the safest possible treatment.

Tip:

Here are examples of medical conditions that are generally considered contraindications for LM after plastic surgery:

1. Active Cancer: While LM can be beneficial for certain cancer patients, particularly those with lymphedema, it may not be suitable for patients with active cancer, especially those with metastasis, due to the risk of potentially spreading the cancer cells.

2. Acute Infections: The lymphatic system plays a key role in fighting infections. Therefore, LM in patients with acute or untreated infections can potentially spread the infectious agents throughout the body.

3. Heart Disease For patients with heart disease or circulatory problems, the increased fluid movement resulting from LM can potentially put strain on the heart. These patients should always consult with their doctor before beginning such therapy.

4. Blood Clots or Thrombophlebitis: LM could potentially dislodge a blood clot, leading to severe complications such as a pulmonary embolism.

5. Kidney Problems: People with severe kidney disease may struggle to process the additional fluid in the body following an LM. This could potentially exacerbate existing kidney issues.

 **LEARN MORE:** Scan or click here to find out what medications may interfere with LM and should be discussed with your healthcare specialist prior to undergoing LM.

34

CAN LYMPHATIC MASSAGE IMPROVE THE APPEARANCE OF CELLULITE AFTER LIPOSUCTION?

Yes, LM can contribute to improving the appearance of cellulite after liposuction. Cellulite occurs when fat cells accumulate and push against the skin while the fibrous tissue bands underneath skin pull it down. This causes a dimpled or "cottage cheese" appearance. LM can help to reduce cellulite by improving lymphatic drainage, which aids in the removal of toxins and waste products from the body, reducing the water retention that can exacerbate the appearance of cellulite.

Furthermore, the massage can help to break up the fibrous tissue bands, resulting in a smoother appearance of the skin. It can also stimulate blood circulation in the area, enhancing skin tone and texture, which can make cellulite less visible. However, it's crucial to remember that while LM can help to reduce the appearance of cellulite, it is not a cure. The effectiveness of the massage in improving cellulite can also depend on various factors, including the individual's skin elasticity, the severity of the cellulite, and adherence to a healthy lifestyle.

Note:

Dry brushing is one of the options to improve cellulite during the later phase of recovery after surgery, when the wounds have fully healed and you can comfortably tolerate more vigorous massage techniques and skin manipulation.

This technique involves brushing the skin with a dry brush and is said to have various benefits for reducing skin cellulite. While the effectiveness may vary from person to person, some potential benefits of dry brushing include:

1. **Exfoliation:** Dry brushing helps to exfoliate the skin by removing dead skin cells and promoting cell turnover. This can lead to smoother and softer skin texture, potentially reducing the appearance of cellulite.

2. **Stimulation of Circulation:** The brushing action of dry brushing can stimulate blood circulation in the targeted areas. Improved circulation may promote the delivery of oxygen and nutrients to the skin, which can help support skin health and potentially reduce the appearance of cellulite.

3. **Lymphatic Drainage:** Dry brushing is often touted as a method to stimulate the lymphatic system, assisting in the removal of toxins and waste products from the body. By promoting lymphatic drainage, it may help reduce fluid retention and swelling, which can contribute to the appearance of cellulite.

4. **Enhanced Absorption of Topical Products:** Dry brushing can create a receptive surface on the skin, potentially enhancing the absorption of topical products, such as cellulite creams or serums, which are applied after brushing.

This may help maximize the benefits of these products in reducing cellulite.

5. **Invigorating and Energizing:** Dry brushing can provide a gentle massage-like sensation, which may promote a sense of invigoration and energy. This can be a refreshing addition to your skincare routine and contribute to overall well-being.

Tip:

Before incorporating dry brushing into your skincare routine, it is essential to obtain permission from your surgeon.

Additionally, discuss with your doctor whether there are any additional topical products that can be recommended to improve skin quality over the surgical sites during the postoperative period. Many plastic surgery offices carry skin products that can be utilized to enhance skin properties after surgery. Do not hesitate to ask for a discount on these products given the recent surgery that you underwent with them.

LEARN MORE:

Scan or click here to learn additional ways to reduce skin cellulite after plastic surgery.

35

How does lymphatic massage enhance the immune system after plastic surgery?

LM can enhance the immune system after plastic surgery through its positive impact on the lymphatic system. The lymphatic system is closely tied to the immune system as it helps remove waste, toxins, and pathogens from the body, while also playing a role in the production and circulation of immune cells. During LM, gentle, rhythmic movements stimulate the flow of lymphatic fluid, assisting in the removal of waste and toxins from the tissues. This process helps to improve the efficiency of the lymphatic system, allowing it to filter and eliminate harmful substances more effectively. By reducing the buildup of waste products and toxins, LM can support the immune system in maintaining optimal function. Furthermore, LM promotes the production and circulation of lymphocytes, a type of white blood cell that plays a crucial role in the immune response. Lymphocytes help identify and destroy pathogens, bacteria, and other foreign substances in the body. By stimulating lymphocyte activity, LM can enhance the immune response, aiding in the body's ability to fight off infections and promote overall wellness.

Note:

Here are some popular natural supplements that are often associated with immune support and may be considered helpful for recovery after plastic surgery.:

1. **Vitamin C:** Known for its immune-boosting properties, vitamin C is an essential nutrient that helps support the immune system. It acts as an antioxidant and plays a vital role in collagen synthesis, which is important for wound healing.

2. **Zinc:** This mineral is involved in various immune functions, including the production and activation of immune cells. Zinc is commonly used to support immune health and promote wound healing.

3. **Vitamin D:** It plays a crucial role in immune regulation and has been associated with improved immune function. Vitamin D can be obtained from sunlight exposure or through dietary supplements.

4. **Probiotics:** These beneficial bacteria support a healthy gut microbiome. They are known to influence immune function positively and may help enhance overall immune response.

5. **Echinacea:** This herb is commonly used for its immune-stimulating properties. It may help support the immune system and shorten the duration and severity of common cold symptoms.

6. **Turmeric:** The active compound in turmeric, called curcumin, has powerful anti-inflammatory and antioxidant

properties. It may help support the immune system and aid in the healing process.

Tip:

Inquire with your surgeon about recommended immune-boosting supplements and the appropriate time to start taking them post-surgery.

LEARN MORE:

Scan or click here to learn about additional ways to boost your immune system after plastic surgery.

36

CAN LYMPHATIC MASSAGE HELP WITH SEROMA PREVENTION OR RESOLUTION AFTER SURGERY?

Yes, LM can be helpful in both prevention and resolution of seromas after surgery. A seroma is a collection of fluid that can accumulate in the surgical area, often due to disrupted lymphatic channels or blood vessels. LM can help address seromas in the following ways:

1. Prevention: By performing LM shortly after surgery, the therapist can help stimulate lymphatic flow and prevent the buildup of fluid. By encouraging proper fluid drainage, LM can help minimize the risk of seroma formation.

2. Resolution: If a seroma has already developed, LM can be used to facilitate its resolution. The gentle techniques employed during the massage help stimulate lymphatic circulation and encourage the drainage of excess fluid from the affected area. This can help to reduce the size of the seroma and promote its absorption by the body.

It's crucial to consult with your healthcare provider or surgeon for personalized advice and guidance on managing seromas after surgery. They can provide specific recommendations and may suggest combining LM with other treatments, such as compression garments or draining procedures, for optimal seroma management.

Note:

After a plastic surgery procedure like abdominoplasty (tummy tuck), a seroma is a potential complication that can develop. A seroma refers to the accumulation of fluid in a space created by surgery, typically in the area where tissue has been removed or repositioned.

During surgery, blood vessels and lymphatic channels can be disrupted, leading to the pooling of lymphatic fluid and blood under the skin. This fluid can collect in a cavity or pocket, resulting in the formation of a seroma. It usually appears as a soft or firm swelling under the skin, often described as a fluid-filled lump or bulge.

Seromas can vary in size and may cause discomfort or pain. They typically occur within the first few weeks after surgery but can develop at any time during the recovery period. Factors that can contribute to the formation of seromas include the extent of tissue dissection, inadequate drainage, trauma to the surgical site, or individual patient factors such as poor tissue healing or excessive physical activity.

In most cases, seromas will resolve on their own as the body reabsorbs the accumulated fluid. However, in some instances, medical intervention may be necessary. Treatment options can include drainage of the seroma with a needle and syringe, the use of compression garments, or in severe cases, surgical intervention.

If you experience signs of a seroma, such as persistent swelling, increased pain, or fluid accumulation, it's important to consult with your healthcare provider or plastic surgeon. They can assess the situation, provide an accurate diagnosis, and recommend appropriate management options tailored to your specific needs.

Tip:

If needle drainage of a seroma is offered at LM therapist's office, it is usually a dangerous sign. Only certified healthcare professionals, such as medical doctors, physician assistants, or trained nurses, are qualified to perform such a procedure. LM therapists are not authorized to perform seroma aspiration unless it is done in a doctor's office under direct supervision. It is always necessary to consult a medical office or hospital for seroma diagnosis and drainage.

LEARN MORE:

Scan or click here to learn more about seroma after plastic surgery and additional ways to prevent seroma formation.

37

CAN LYMPHATIC MASSAGE HELP WITH POSTOPERATIVE EDEMA IN THE EXTREMITIES AFTER SURGERY?

Yes, LM can help with postoperative edema in the extremities after surgery. Increased swelling in the legs can be a result of several factors specific to plastic surgery. First, significant tissue trauma from procedures such as liposuction or abdominoplasty may lead to partial destruction of functioning lymphatic pathways, resulting in fluid accumulation below the level of the trauma. In the case of abdominoplasty, the incision in the lower abdomen can disrupt lymphatic vessels that normally provide drainage from a large area, including the lower extremities. This disruption can contribute to persistent lower leg edema. Additionally, flank liposuction may further disrupt lymphatic drainage as collateral lymphatic vessels can also be affected by the trauma to the soft tissue.

Low mobility can also result in reduced function of the natural muscle pump mechanism in the lower legs, leading to fluid accumulation. Prolonged sitting with flexed legs, particularly after abdominoplasty, can create additional resistance for the transfer of edema fluid into the lymphatic collectors, resulting in increased edema. Finally, the use of high body compression garments, such as abdominal binders, fajas, or abdominal boards, may constrict or obstruct the residual functioning lymphatic vessels, leading to more severe fluid accumulation below the level of compression.

Incorporating LM into the postoperative care plan can help stimulate lymphatic flow, improve circulation, and facilitate the drainage of excess fluid from the affected extremities.

Note:

Although swelling in both legs may be a result of decreased lymphatic flow, if you encounter this, it is important to discuss it with your surgeon. Severe leg swelling can indicate the presence of serious complications. If you experience asymmetric leg swelling, with one leg significantly bigger than the other, it is crucial to communicate with your surgeon promptly, as it can be a sign of a dangerous complication such as blood clots.

Avoid requesting diuretics or water pills from your doctor to reduce leg swelling without proper consultation. It is important to discuss any leg swelling during the recovery period with your doctor and have it examined. Your doctor will be able to provide appropriate guidance and determine the underlying cause of the swelling to ensure the most suitable approach.

Tip:

Use a measuring tape to determine the circumference of your lower leg close to the ankle joint. It is recommended to record this measurement weekly to track and evaluate the progress in reducing swelling after surgery. This can help you monitor changes in the swelling and assess the effectiveness of LM.

LEARN MORE:

Scan or click <u>here</u> to learn how to reduce body swelling after plastic surgery.

38

IS LYMPHATIC MASSAGE APPROPRIATE FOR EVERY KIND OF PLASTIC SURGERY PROCEDURE?

LM can be beneficial for many types of plastic surgery procedures. It is commonly used after procedures such as liposuction, abdominoplasty (tummy tuck), breast augmentation or reduction, facelift, and body contouring surgeries. However, it is important to note that the suitability of LM may vary depending on individual factors and the specific details of the surgery.

For most procedures, LM is typically recommended and considered an integral part of the postoperative care plan. It can help promote healing, reduce swelling and inflammation, improve lymphatic flow, and enhance overall recovery. Your surgeon or healthcare provider can advise you on whether LM is appropriate for your specific procedure and guide you on the optimal timing and frequency of the massages.

Note:

Some of the common procedures where LM is often recommended include:

1. Liposuction: LM can help reduce postoperative swelling, improve lymphatic drainage, and promote smoother healing after liposuction. In combination with light deep tissue techniques it can decrease fibrosis in soft tissue.

2. Abdominoplasty (Tummy Tuck): LM can aid in reducing swelling and fluid retention in the abdominal area, assisting with postoperative healing and contouring.

3. Breast Augmentation or Reduction: LM can help alleviate swelling, promote lymphatic flow, and enhance the healing process after breast surgery.

4. Facelift: LM can assist in reducing postoperative swelling, promoting lymphatic drainage, and enhancing overall facial rejuvenation after a facelift procedure.

5. Body Contouring Surgeries: Procedures such as body lifts, thigh lifts, or arm lifts can benefit from LM to reduce swelling, promote healing, and improve the overall outcome.

Tip:

LM is more commonly sought after body procedures, particularly liposuction. However, it is less frequently performed after cosmetic procedures such as facelifts or breast surgery, despite the evident benefits. If you are considering LM after a facelift or breast surgery, it is essential to inquire about your LM therapist's experience with these specific surgeries. Ask them directly about their level of expertise and experience in providing LM for face and breast procedures. This will help ensure that you receive the appropriate care and guidance tailored to your specific needs.

LEARN MORE:

Scan or click here to learn about specific plastic surgery procedures or conditions where LM needs to be performed with special caution after it's approved by your surgeon.

39

CAN LYMPHATIC MASSAGE AID IN THE RESOLUTION OF A HEMATOMA AFTER PLASTIC SURGERY?

LM may have a limited role in aiding the resolution of a hematoma after plastic surgery. A hematoma is a collection of blood that forms outside of blood vessels, typically due to bleeding during or after a surgical procedure.

In the early stages of hematoma formation, the focus is usually on managing the hematoma itself through techniques such as compression, drainage, or surgical intervention. LM, with its gentle manual techniques, may not directly address the hematoma but can indirectly assist with the healing process.

LM can help improve lymphatic circulation and stimulate the drainage of excess fluid from the affected area. By reducing swelling and promoting lymphatic flow, it may help enhance the body's natural healing mechanisms and potentially contribute to the resolution of the hematoma over time.

Note:

After an abdominoplasty procedure, a hematoma can form in the surgical area. It occurs when a collection of blood vessels are damaged during the surgery, leading to bleeding that accumulates under the skin or in the deeper tissues. Hematomas can vary in size and severity, ranging from small, localized areas to larger, more extensive collections of blood.

Signs and symptoms of a hematoma after abdominoplasty may include swelling, bruising, and increased pain, or discomfort in the surgical area. The hematoma may feel firm or tender to the touch. In some cases, a hematoma can cause additional complications, such as increased risk of infection or delayed wound healing. If a hematoma is suspected or diagnosed after abdominoplasty, it is important to consult with your surgeon or healthcare provider. They will evaluate the extent of the hematoma and may recommend appropriate management options, such as observation, drainage, or surgical intervention. Treatment for a hematoma typically involves addressing the underlying cause of the bleeding and ensuring proper wound healing.

Tip:

Bromelain, an enzyme found in pineapple, has been studied for its potential to reduce a hematoma after surgery. Although there is some evidence suggesting its benefits, the research is limited, and the results are not conclusive. Bromelain is believed to have anti-inflammatory properties, which may help reduce swelling and inflammation associated with a hematoma. It is thought to work by inhibiting certain inflammatory molecules in the body. Additionally, bromelain has been suggested to have fibrinolytic activity, meaning it can help break down fibrin, a protein involved in blood clot formation.

While some studies have shown promising results in reducing postoperative edema and inflammation with bromelain supplementation, more research is needed to establish its effectiveness specifically for hematoma reduction. It is important to note that individual responses to bromelain may vary, and it should always be used under the guidance and recommendation of a healthcare professional.

LEARN MORE:

Scan or click here to learn about additional ways to decrease risk of hematoma.

40

How does lymphatic massage contribute to overall well-being and relaxation during the recovery period?

LM can contribute to overall well-being and relaxation during the recovery period in several ways:

1. Stress reduction: The gentle and rhythmic strokes of LM promote relaxation by activating the parasympathetic nervous system, which helps counteract the body's stress response. This can lead to a reduction in anxiety, tension, and overall stress levels, promoting a sense of calm and well-being.

2. Improved sleep quality: LM has been reported to improve sleep quality in individuals recovering from surgery. By reducing pain, promoting relaxation, and enhancing circulation, it can contribute to better sleep patterns and more restorative rest during the recovery period.

3. Enhanced mood and mental well-being: LM stimulates the release of endorphins, the body's natural "feel-good" chemicals. This can result in an uplifted mood, decreased feelings of depression or anxiety, and an overall sense of well-being. The therapeutic touch of the massage therapist can also provide emotional support and create a nurturing environment for relaxation and healing.

4. Increased body awareness: LM can help individuals become more attuned to their bodies during the recovery period. By focusing on the new sensations and responses of the body, it promotes a deeper connection and understanding of the healing process. This increased body awareness can empower individuals to take an active role in their recovery, make informed decisions, and practice self-care.

5. Promotes lymphatic flow and detoxification: LM specifically targets the lymphatic system, promoting the circulation and drainage of lymph fluid. This helps to remove metabolic waste, toxins, and excess fluid from the tissues, supporting the body's natural detoxification processes. By enhancing lymphatic flow, LM can contribute to a sense of lightness, improved energy levels, and overall well-being.

It is important to note that individual experiences may vary, and the benefits of LM during the recovery period can be influenced by factors such as the specific procedure, overall health, and individual response to the massage. Consulting with a certified and experienced LM therapist can help tailor the massage sessions to your specific needs and enhance overall well-being and relaxation during the recovery period.

Note:

Aromatherapy plays a significant role in promoting overall well-being and relaxation. It is a holistic practice that involves using natural plant extracts, known as essential oils, to enhance physical, emotional, and mental health. The aromas of these essential oils have a direct impact on the limbic system, the part of the brain responsible for emotions and memories, triggering various responses in the body.

In terms of relaxation, specific essential oils like lavender, chamomile, and ylang-ylang are known for their calming properties, reducing stress, anxiety, and promoting better sleep quality. The gentle, soothing scents can create a tranquil ambiance in a room or during massage sessions, facilitating a sense of calmness and relaxation.

Beyond relaxation, aromatherapy can contribute to overall well-being by addressing specific health concerns. Essential oils like eucalyptus, peppermint, and tea tree have potential therapeutic benefits for respiratory health and immune support. Others, such as rosemary and lemon, can promote focus and mental clarity.

Aromatherapy can be incorporated into various practices like massage therapy, meditation, or even as part of daily self-care routines. Whether diffused in the air, applied topically, or used in baths, the aromatic experience of essential oils can positively impact both physical and emotional states, fostering a sense of harmony and balance in the body and mind. It is essential to choose high-quality essential oils and use them responsibly to fully enjoy the benefits of aromatherapy for overall well-being and relaxation.

Tip:

Ask your LM therapist about techniques for stress reduction you can utilize at home.

There are several techniques to reduce stress while recovering from plastic surgery. Here are some effective strategies:

1. **Deep breathing exercises:** This is a simple yet powerful technique to calm the nervous system and reduce stress. Practice slow, deep breaths, inhaling deeply through your nose and exhaling slowly through your mouth. Focus on the sensation of the breath entering and leaving your body, allowing your mind to become more centered and relaxed.

2. **Meditation and mindfulness:** Engaging in meditation or mindfulness practices can help alleviate stress and promote a sense of inner calm. Find a quiet and comfortable space, close your eyes, and focus on the present moment. You can use guided meditation apps or follow breathing techniques to guide your practice and cultivate a peaceful state of mind.

3. **Gentle stretching and yoga:** Once approved by your surgeon, engaging in gentle stretching exercises or practicing yoga can help release tension in the body and promote relaxation. Choose gentle postures and movements that feel comfortable for your healing body. Pay attention to your body's limits and avoid any poses that cause discomfort or strain.

4. **Engage in enjoyable activities:** Find activities that bring you joy and help you relax. This can include reading a book, listening to soothing music, watching a favorite movie or TV show, practicing a hobby, or spending time with loved ones. Engaging in activities that bring you happiness can divert your focus from stress and promote emotional well-being.

5. **Seek support:** Reach out to family, friends, or support groups who can provide emotional support during your recovery. Sharing your concerns, fears, or feelings with

others who understand and empathize can help alleviate stress. Professional support from a therapist or counselor can also be beneficial in managing stress and promoting emotional well-being during the recovery process.

6. **Adequate Sleep:** Aim for seven to ten hours of sleep each night for optimal healing. Quality of sleep is crucial, especially during the initial recovery phase when your body demands more rest, both day and night. This period is vital for healing, as the body uses stored energy and naturally induces fatigue to aid recovery. Plan for and embrace this natural process by arranging comfortable sleep in a quiet environment.

7. **Talk Therapy:** Sharing your surgery experience can be therapeutic. Connecting with friends or family who have undergone similar procedures can be immensely comforting, offering a sense of camaraderie, an understanding of the surgery and recovery process, and support working through the accompanying emotions. If your surgical experience was challenging, seeking a professional counselor might be beneficial. They can assist you in processing your experience and emotions, helping to restore a sense of acceptance and tranquility.

LEARN MORE: Scan or click here to learn how to enhance your mental health after plastic surgery.

41

WHAT ARE THE SIGNS THAT ADDITIONAL LYMPHATIC MASSAGE SESSIONS ARE NECESSARY AFTER PLASTIC SURGERY?

There are several signs that may indicate the need for additional LM sessions after plastic surgery. It is important to listen to your body and communicate with your LM therapist and surgeon to determine the best course of action. Here are some signs to be aware of:

1. **Persistent swelling:** While some degree of swelling is normal after surgery, if you notice that the swelling persists or worsens over time, it may indicate the need for additional LM sessions. LM can help promote lymphatic drainage and reduce excess fluid buildup in the tissues.

2. **Limited range of motion:** If you experience limited range of motion in the affected area, such as difficulty moving a joint or performing certain movements, it may indicate the presence of fibrosis or adhesions. LM and light deep tissue

massage can help break down these adhesions and improve mobility.

3. **Increased discomfort or pain:** If you notice an increase in discomfort or pain in the surgical area, it could be a sign of inflammation, tension, or congestion. LM can help alleviate these symptoms by reducing inflammation, promoting circulation, and releasing muscle tension.

4. **Uneven or asymmetrical appearance:** If you notice an asymmetry or unevenness in the treated area, it may indicate the need for additional LM sessions. LM can help address any fluid imbalances, promote even healing, and improve the overall aesthetic outcome.

5. **Slow healing or delayed recovery:** If you feel that your recovery process is taking longer than expected or if you are not progressing as anticipated, it may be beneficial to consider additional LM sessions. LM can support the body's natural healing processes and help expedite the recovery timeline.

Note:

If you have undergone surgery and are considering LM, it is best to consult with an LM specialist to determine if it would be beneficial for you. In general, LM can be beneficial for most individuals after surgery. Your LM therapist will assess your recovery progress and provide guidance on the recommended number of additional LM sessions for optimal results.

Tip:

If, during the early stages of your recovery, you missed the opportunity to incorporate LM and are now you want to try it to help aid your recovery, rest assured that it's not too late. Lymphatic

Massage can still play a crucial role in enhancing your healing, even if you're in the more advanced phases of recovery.

 **LEARN MORE:** Scan or click here to learn more about the effects of LM during different post-surgical recovery phases.

42

IS LYMPHATIC MASSAGE RECOMMENDED FOR PATIENTS WHO UNDERGO MULTIPLE PROCEDURES SIMULTANEOUSLY?

LM may be helpful for patients who undergo multiple procedures simultaneously, but it is important to consult with your surgeon and LM therapist to determine the most appropriate approach for your specific case. The decision to undergo LM after multiple procedures will depend on factors such as the extent of the surgeries, the overall health and healing capacity of the individual, and any specific considerations related to the procedures performed.

In some cases, it may be advisable to delay LM until a certain point in the recovery process to ensure that the body has had sufficient time to heal and stabilize. This allows for a more targeted and tailored approach to the LM sessions based on the specific areas treated during the multiple procedures.

Note:

LM after multiple plastic surgical procedures can pose greater challenges for LM therapists and requires a higher level of expertise. The presence of multiple incisions and surgical sites can lead to more significant disruption of the lymphatic flow. LM therapists need to possess extensive knowledge of anatomy, physiology, and pathophysiology to recognize residual and accessory lymphatic pathways and adjust their techniques accordingly to facilitate lymphatic drainage in these complex cases.

Tip:

If you are seeking an LM therapist to perform LM after undergoing multiple simultaneous cosmetic body procedures, the best recommendation is to book an appointment with the most experienced specialist available.

LM following multiple simultaneous surgical procedures necessitates a longer treatment duration to thoroughly address all the affected areas. Such LM sessions may extend to 90 minutes, as opposed to the more traditional 60-minute session, to ensure comprehensive coverage and effective treatment across all surgical sites.

 **LEARN MORE:**

Scan or click here to learn more about LM after multiple plastic surgeries.

43

WHAT IS THE ROLE OF LYMPHATIC MASSAGE IN REDUCING POSTOPERATIVE BRUISING AND DISCOLORATION?

The role of LM in reducing postoperative bruising and discoloration is multifaceted and plays a significant role in enhancing the body's natural healing processes. Following surgery, the body often experiences accumulation of small blood clots and particles in the soft tissues, manifesting as visible bruises on the skin. The body naturally mobilizes specific cells designed to eliminate these particles, and LM can expedite this process:

1. **Increased Blood Flow:** Mechanical stimulation from LM increases blood flow to the bruised areas. This increased circulation delivers more cells to the region, thereby facilitating the resolution of bruising more rapidly.

2. **Fluid Reduction:** After surgery, excessive fluid or swelling is a common occurrence. LM aids in the elimination of this excess

fluid, making it easier for the body's natural processes to absorb the bruises.

3. **Inflammation Reduction:** LM can help to reduce inflammation in the surgical site. Decreased inflammation aids in the body's reparative processes, contributing to faster bruising improvement.

4. **Toxin and Waste Removal:** By stimulating the lymphatic system, massage aids in the elimination of toxins and blood particles, which can expedite bruise healing. This is achieved by reducing local inflammation and facilitating the clearing process of the affected tissues.

Note:

In addition to LM and the use of post-surgical compression garments, several other methods can be employed to decrease bruising following plastic surgery. Nutritional supplements, such as bromelain and arnica montana, have been shown to aid postoperative recovery. Bromelain, derived from pineapples, possesses anti-inflammatory and anti-swelling properties, potentially accelerating the healing process. Similarly, arnica montana, a plant native to Europe, has been used in homeopathic medicine for centuries to reduce bruising and swelling. Outside of supplements, ensuring adequate hydration, maintaining a nutritious diet rich in vitamins (especially Vitamin C and K), and abstaining from substances that can increase bleeding, like alcohol and certain medications, can further promote healing. Rest and elevation of the affected area can also significantly reduce swelling and speed up recovery.

Tip:

Speak with your physician or lymphatic massage therapist to determine which supplements for reducing bruising might be most suitable for your unique circumstances.

LEARN MORE:

Scan or click here to learn about the top ten natural anti-bruising agents.

44

CAN LYMPHATIC MASSAGE HELP WITH POSTOPERATIVE NUMBNESS OR HYPERSENSITIVITY IN THE SURGICAL AREAS?

Yes, LM can potentially help with postoperative numbness and hypersensitivity in surgical areas. After surgery, numbness and hypersensitivity may occur due to nerve irritation or damage, inflammation, or the body's natural response to trauma. Here's how LM can help:

1. **Promotes Nerve Regeneration:** Gentle stimulation through massage can help awaken and encourage regeneration of damaged or traumatized nerves, thereby reducing numbness.

2. **Reduces Inflammation and Swelling:** By stimulating the lymphatic system and promoting fluid drainage, LM can help to reduce inflammation and swelling. These are common causes of nerve compression, which can lead to symptoms like numbness and hypersensitivity. By reducing swelling

116

and inflammation, pressure on the nerves can be relieved, improving these symptoms.

3. **Improves Circulation:** LM can enhance circulation in the treated area, delivering more oxygen and nutrients that are necessary for nerve healing and reducing symptoms of numbness and hypersensitivity.

4. **Alleviates Pain and Hypersensitivity:** The gentle pressure and rhythmic movements of LM can soothe hypersensitive areas, providing relief from discomfort and pain.

However, it's important to remember that while LM can be beneficial for these symptoms, it may not be suitable for everyone and is not the only treatment option. It's essential to consult a healthcare provider before starting LM to ensure it is appropriate for your specific situation and is not going to interfere with your healing process or cause further issues. Additionally, any persistent numbness or hypersensitivity should be reported to your healthcare provider, as it may be a sign of a more serious issue that needs to be addressed.

Note:

Experiencing alterations in sensation at the surgery site is a relatively common occurrence and can be either temporary or permanent. The process of nerve regeneration after surgery is usually slow and can take from several months up to a year. It's crucial for you to pay close attention to any changes in sensitivity, whether they involve numbness or heightened sensitivity. Make sure to keep both your doctor and your LM therapist informed about these changes. They can guide you and adjust your treatment plan accordingly to aid your healing process.

Tip:

During your body's recovery period after surgery, you might notice temporary changes in skin sensitivity. Be cautious when using heating or cooling pads or devices. Due to decreased skin sensitivity, you could inadvertently cause significant tissue damage through prolonged application of heat or cold to these less sensitive areas. It's always crucial to seek advice from a healthcare professional before using such devices to ensure safe and appropriate use.

LEARN MORE:

Scan or click here to understand more about changes in sensitivity and learn tips to facilitate nerve recovery.

45

WHAT ARE THE KEY DIFFERENCES BETWEEN PROFESSIONAL LYMPHATIC MASSAGE AND SELF-PERFORMED LYMPHATIC DRAINAGE TECHNIQUES?

Professional LM and self-performed lymphatic drainage techniques share the same goal of stimulating the lymphatic system to remove waste and toxins, reduce inflammation, and improve circulation. However, they differ significantly in terms of technique, efficacy, and safety.

A professional LM is performed by a certified therapist who has undergone extensive training to understand the anatomy and physiology of the lymphatic system. They know the precise techniques to stimulate lymph flow without causing injury or discomfort, and they can adapt their methods based on individual patient needs. Furthermore, a professional can target deep lymph nodes and vessels that are hard to reach or require specialized techniques. They can also provide a more comprehensive treatment, addressing the entire body's lymphatic system rather than just localized areas.

In contrast, self-performed lymphatic drainage techniques, though convenient and cost-effective, have certain limitations. Unless guided by a professional, these techniques may not be executed correctly, potentially leading to ineffective treatment or, in some cases, harm. The techniques that individuals can safely and effectively perform on themselves generally only target superficial lymph nodes and vessels and may not stimulate the lymphatic system as effectively as a professional massage. Also, self-performed techniques tend to focus on localized areas and may not adequately address the whole lymphatic system.

Note:

While both professional LM and self-performed lymphatic drainage techniques can aid in stimulating the lymphatic system, a professional massage is typically more effective and comprehensive, thanks to the therapist's specialized training and knowledge. However, self-performed techniques can be a useful supplement to professional treatment, especially when guided by a professional, and they provide a convenient, accessible, and cost-effective option for regular lymphatic stimulation. It's always important to consult a healthcare provider before starting any new health regimen to ensure it's suitable and safe.

Tip:

Consider asking your LM therapist to show you particular techniques that you could apply at home to aid in your recovery.

LEARN MORE:

Scan or click <u>here</u> to learn more about the advantages and drawbacks of professional and self-administered LM.

46

IS LYMPHATIC MASSAGE SUITABLE FOR PATIENTS WITH CHRONIC PAIN CONDITIONS WHO UNDERGO PLASTIC SURGERY?

LM may be beneficial for patients with chronic pain conditions who undergo plastic surgery, but it's critical that this decision is made on an individual basis, in consultation with healthcare providers.

Chronic pain conditions can be complex, and the effects of LM will depend on the specifics of the condition. In some cases, the gentle, rhythmic movements of LM can help alleviate pain and discomfort by reducing inflammation, promoting circulation, and supporting the body's natural healing processes. This can be particularly beneficial after surgery, where these processes can help manage postoperative swelling, bruising, and discomfort.

However, it's important to note that some chronic pain conditions may make patients more sensitive to touch or pressure, which could potentially make LM uncomfortable. In other instances, certain chronic pain conditions might be exacerbated by massage.

Note:

The interaction between plastic surgery and chronic pain conditions can be complex, and how a patient's chronic pain will affect their surgical recovery is highly individual. Therefore, it's crucial that any decision about LM or other postoperative care be made in close consultation with the patient's healthcare providers. They can consider the specifics of the patient's condition, their overall health, the nature of their surgery, and their personal preferences to make recommendations that will be both safe and beneficial.

Tip:

It's crucial to always share your full medical history, including any chronic conditions, with both your surgeon and your LM therapist. This information helps them plan the best approach for your treatment and recovery. Don't hesitate to ask your LM therapist about the various massage techniques they can use to assist in your recovery after plastic surgery, especially those that might be particularly beneficial for managing your chronic conditions.

LEARN MORE:

Scan or click here to learn about the top ten chronic health conditions where LM can be beneficial.

47

CAN LYMPHATIC MASSAGE BE PERFORMED ON PATIENTS WITH OPEN WOUNDS OR ACTIVE INFECTIONS?

LM should generally not be performed on patients with open wounds or active infections. This is primarily for two reasons:

1. **Risk of exacerbating the condition or spreading infection:** LM stimulates the flow of lymph, which carries substances throughout the body. If an infection is present, there's a risk that the massage could potentially spread the infection to other parts of the body. Similarly, massaging an area with an open wound could disrupt the healing process and exacerbate the condition.

2. **Risk of injury and discomfort:** Massage on or near an open wound or active infection can be painful and could potentially cause further injury. It's critical to allow the body time to heal properly before engaging in massage therapy.

However, in some cases, a modified form of LM may be performed to aid healing by reducing nearby swelling and improving circulation, but this should be done only under the guidance of a trained healthcare professional and not directly on the open wound or infected area.

Note:

An expert LM therapist will always let you know if there are healing issues at your surgical sites that might mean you need to delay your LM session. It's essential to also check with your surgeon, to ask whether you should continue with the massages or pause them, and if so, for how long. If an LM therapist overlooks an open wound or possible infection, that could be a warning sign. In such cases, it might be worth seeking a second opinion from another LM specialist. Your health and safety should always be the top priority.

Tip:

1. If you're worried about potential complications at your surgical site that might make LM unsuitable, it's vital to reach out to both your surgeon and your LM therapist. To help them assess the situation without you needing to make a potentially unnecessary trip, you could consider taking a photo of the area you're worried about and sending it to them for review. They can then provide advice based on their expert evaluation of the situation. Your health and safety should always come first.

2. Inquire whether your LM therapist performs LM on clients with post-surgical wounds. If so, ensure that the therapist adheres to the highest standards of antiseptic cleaning for both their hands and equipment to avoid cross-contamination.

LEARN MORE:

Scan or click <u>here</u> to learn more about navigating LM with a post-surgical wound.

48

IS LYMPHATIC MASSAGE BENEFICIAL FOR PATIENTS WHO UNDERGO GENDER-AFFIRMING SURGERIES?

Yes, LM can be beneficial for patients who undergo gender-affirming surgeries, such as top surgery or genital reconstruction surgery. These procedures can lead to post-operative swelling, bruising, and discomfort, all of which may be alleviated by LM.

1. **Reduction of Swelling:** LM helps to stimulate the lymphatic system, which can reduce post-surgical swelling and bruising. This can improve comfort and potentially speed up the healing process.

2. **Pain Relief:** The gentle, rhythmic movements of LM can help alleviate postoperative pain and discomfort, contributing to a more comfortable recovery process.

3. **Improved Healing:** By enhancing the circulation of lymphatic fluid, LM can help to remove waste products and

toxins from the body and bring essential nutrients to healing tissues, which can promote faster and more effective healing.

4. **Scar Tissue Management:** Regular LM might help to soften and break down scar tissue over time, potentially improving the cosmetic outcome of surgery.

Note:

LM can play a pivotal role in the recovery process following top surgery. By assisting in the reduction of swelling, it helps in promoting a more refined chest and breast contour. Additionally, the gentle manipulation during the massage can aid in minimizing scarring, providing a smoother appearance over time. Moreover, LM can significantly lessen the risk of seroma formation, which is a collection of fluid that can occur after surgery, by enhancing fluid drainage and encouraging proper lymphatic function. Thus, incorporating LM into your post-operative care routine can be a holistic approach to facilitate healing and achieve desired surgical outcomes.

Tip:

Gender-affirming surgeries often involve more intricate procedures compared to typical plastic surgery, and as such, it's beneficial if your LM therapist is well-versed in the specialized techniques required post-operatively. This ensures they can provide the most appropriate and effective care for your unique needs following such procedures. Consider asking whether the prospective LM therapist is familiar with LM techniques specifically for genre affirming surgery.

LEARN MORE:

Scan or click here to find out more about specific LM techniques after gender-affirming mastectomy surgery.

49

IS LYMPHATIC MASSAGE SUITABLE FOR PATIENTS WITH A HISTORY OF ALLERGIES OR SENSITIVITIES TO SKINCARE PRODUCTS?

LM can generally be safely performed on patients with a history of allergies or sensitivities to skincare products. The main consideration here is that the massage therapist should be made aware of these sensitivities prior to the treatment to ensure that they do not use any oils, lotions, or other products that could trigger an allergic reaction or skin sensitivity.

The techniques used for LM do not typically involve the use of many skincare products, focusing instead on gentle, rhythmic movements to stimulate the flow of lymph. However, some therapists might use specific lotions or oils to facilitate their movements on the skin. Therefore, clear communication about any known allergies or sensitivities is essential to avoid any adverse reactions.

If the patient has a history of severe allergic reactions, such as anaphylaxis, or if they have highly sensitive skin, it may be advisable to perform a patch test with any proposed products before the massage. This involves applying a small amount of the product to a discrete area of skin to confirm there is no reaction.

In conclusion, while LM can generally be performed on those with allergies or sensitivities to skincare products, it's crucial to ensure that your therapist is aware of these conditions. This ensures that your treatment is not only effective but also safe and comfortable.

Note:

While your LM therapist might use oils to help with their techniques, it's essential to check that you don't have any allergies to the components of these oils, even though such allergies are relatively rare. It's always better to err on the side of caution to ensure your massage is not just beneficial, but also safe for your skin.

Tip:

If you have allergies to certain substances commonly found in skincare products, it's wise to check the ingredients of any topical products your LM therapist plans to use during your session. Be sure to do this for every appointment and with each new therapist you see. This proactive approach helps ensure your sessions are both beneficial and safe, avoiding any adverse reactions.

LEARN MORE:

Scan or click here to learn more about benefits of LM for your skin.

50

ARE THERE ANY RESTRICTIONS OR LIMITATIONS ON ACTIVITIES OR MOVEMENTS FOLLOWING LYMPHATIC MASSAGE AFTER PLASTIC SURGERY?

Yes, there can be some restrictions or limitations on activities and movements following LM after plastic surgery, primarily for the purpose of protecting the surgical site and promoting healing. However, these will depend on the specifics of your surgery, the area of your body that was operated on, and your overall health. Here are a few general guidelines:

1. **Avoid Strenuous Activities:** Right after an LM session, it's generally advised to avoid strenuous physical activities like heavy lifting or intense exercise.

2. **Careful Movement:** Especially if you've had surgery in an area that's involved in movement (like joints, or abdominal area with a tummy tuck, you'll need to be careful about how

you move to avoid putting stress on the surgical site. Your healthcare provider can give you specific guidance on what movements to avoid.

3. **Wear Compression Garments:** If your healthcare provider has recommended wearing compression garments after your surgery, it's important to continue doing so after your LM appointment. These garments can help reduce swelling and support healing.

4. **Stay Hydrated and Rest:** Hydration is crucial for lymphatic function and overall recovery. After you LM, make sure to drink plenty of water to help flush the excess fluid and toxins from your body. Also, ensure you get plenty of rest to allow your body to heal.

Note:

Remember that these are general guidelines and might not apply to everyone. Always consult your healthcare provider or your LM therapist for personalized advice based on your specific circumstances. They can provide recommendations tailored to your needs to ensure a safe and effective recovery.

Tip:

If you're ever uncertain, don't hesitate to ask your LM therapist if there are any restrictions on physical activity after each session. It's important to know what you can and can't do to ensure a safe and effective recovery process.

LEARN MORE:

Scan or click here to learn about recommendations for activity after LM.

51

IS LYMPHATIC MASSAGE PAINFUL?

LM after plastic surgery, when conducted by a certified and experienced therapist, is designed to be a gentle and soothing experience. The technique involves light, rhythmic strokes to stimulate the lymphatic system, and does not involve the deep or rigorous pressure that might be associated with other forms of massage, especially deep tissue. The goal is to ease the body into better health, not cause additional discomfort.

It's important to note that while LM should never cause pain, some minor discomfort might be experienced during the early stages of recovery. This can be due to the body's natural reaction to surgery and should not be confused with the massage being painful. Any discomfort experienced should be mild, generally not exceeding a two or three on a pain scale from one to ten, where one signifies no pain and ten signifies the worst pain imaginable.

Effective communication with your LM therapist is crucial to ensure that the pressure during the massage remains within your comfort zone. Pain can cause muscle and vascular spasms which can lead to more fluid retention, potentially slowing down the recovery process. If you ever experience discomfort beyond what you feel is acceptable, it's important to immediately inform your therapist so they can adjust their techniques accordingly. Remember, your comfort and well-being are paramount during this recovery journey.

Note:

There are several strategies that many LM therapists recommend to decrease discomfort during LM sessions. These typically focus on optimizing the conditions for manual stimulation. For example, ensuring a comfortable room temperature, using an electrical and soft foam massage table, and employing gentle, soothing music can all help create a relaxing environment conducive to healing.

In addition, some therapists may suggest the use of topical pain creams and lotions. These can help numb the skin surface and provide a more comfortable massage experience. Please consult with your therapist regarding specific products that they might recommend.

The use of over-the-counter pain medication, such as acetaminophen or ibuprofen, prior to an LM session is a matter of professional discretion and patient preference. While these medications can help manage discomfort, their use should be considered cautiously due to potential side effects and interactions with other post-surgical medications. Always consult with your surgeon or a medical professional before adding any new medication to your regimen.

Tip:

Consider employing mindful breathing techniques during your session. This can help you relax and may make the experience more enjoyable. Remember, communication is key—always let your therapist know if you're experiencing discomfort so they can adjust their technique accordingly. This will help ensure that your LM is a beneficial part of your recovery, rather than a source of additional stress or pain.

LEARN MORE:

Scan or click <u>here</u> for tips on pain reduction during LM.

52

WHAT ARE THE SIGNS THAT LYMPHATIC MASSAGE IS WORKING? HOW DO I KNOW THAT LYMPHATIC IS HELPING?

Determining the effectiveness of LM after a surgical procedure can sometimes be subjective, as each individual's body responds differently to the treatment. However, there are certain indicators that can suggest the massage is doing its intended job:

1. **Reduced Swelling:** One of the primary goals of LM is to reduce swelling by promoting the flow of lymphatic fluid away from congested areas. If you notice a decrease in puffiness or swelling in the area where the massage was performed, this is a positive sign that the massage is working.

2. **Decreased Pain and Discomfort:** Many people report that LM can help alleviate pain and discomfort following surgery. If you experience less pain in the days following your massage, it might be an indication that the therapy is beneficial.

3. **Improved Mobility:** With reduced swelling and pain, you might find your range of motion improves. This can be a good sign that the LM is facilitating your healing process. It is not uncommon to notice enhanced mobility and an improvement in posture following an initial LM treatment.

4. **Faster Healing:** If your surgical wounds seem to be healing faster, with less redness, bruising or heat around the area, this may be another sign that the LM is aiding in your recovery.

5. **General Well-being:** Many patients report feeling more relaxed and having an overall sense of well-being after LMs. Stress reduction can be a significant component in the healing process.

Note:

Increased urination following an LM is a common physiological reaction, resulting from the improved circulation and processing of bodily fluids. This can serve as an indicator of the effectiveness of LM.

During LM, the therapist uses light, rhythmic strokes to stimulate the lymphatic system, a network of tissues and organs that helps rid the body of toxins, waste, and other unwanted materials. The primary function of the lymphatic system is to transport lymph, a fluid containing infection-fighting white blood cells, throughout the body.

When lymphatic circulation is improved through massage, excess fluid from the tissues is moved into the lymphatic vessels and then returned to the bloodstream. From here, these fluids —which may include toxins, waste products, and excess water—are transported to the kidneys.

The kidneys play a vital role in filtering the blood and removing waste products through the production of urine. Therefore, when the lymphatic system is stimulated through massage, and more fluid is being processed by the body, it can result in an increased production of urine as the body expels these excess fluids and waste.

This increase in urination is one of the signs that the LM is effectively helping your body to eliminate waste products and reduce swelling and inflammation. However, if you have any concerns about any changes in your urination, you should discuss them with your healthcare provider.

Tip:

1. Following LM, your body may need additional hydration due to increased urination. It's important to replenish your body's fluids with high-quality water, or a beverage of your preference. Optimal hydration is key to ensuring a smooth recovery after plastic surgery.

2. It's advisable to empty any surgical drains you may have before your massage session, as this will allow you to visually observe the increased lymph flow following the massage. Consider taking a picture before and after the massage session to potentially notice the difference. If you are wearing a compression garment, does it become easier to fasten, and do you find it becoming looser after a few sessions? This could be a tangible sign of reduced swelling and improved lymphatic drainage.

LEARN MORE:

Scan or click here to learn about ways to measure reduction of swelling after LM.

53

IS IT POSSIBLE TO EXPERIENCE DISCOMFORT OR FEEL UNWELL FOLLOWING LYMPHATIC DRAINAGE?

While it's relatively rare, some individuals may experience slight discomfort following an LM. This temporary sensation is often linked to the body's accelerated elimination of waste products. LM activates the lymphatic system, which plays a crucial role in expelling toxins and waste from the body. The massage technique enhances lymph flow, thereby aiding in more efficient waste removal.

However, for those not accustomed to this heightened detoxification rate, the body might respond with symptoms resembling mild sickness. These symptoms can include slight nausea, feelings of fatigue, or experiencing lightheadedness and occasional headaches. This reaction is sometimes termed a "healing crisis" or a "detox reaction."

To alleviate these symptoms, it's recommended to hydrate adequately before and after an LM, aiding in the more effective flushing out of toxins. Furthermore, engaging in rest and light activities such as walking can assist your body in adapting to these changes.

Should you consistently experience discomfort following LM sessions, or if your symptoms are intense or linger beyond a couple of days, seeking advice from a healthcare professional is crucial. They can eliminate other potential causes and offer advice on managing your symptoms effectively.

Note:

As your body heals after surgery, its ability to process and eliminate toxins improves, a function that LM can further enhance. Therefore, even if you initially encounter discomfort akin to a "detox crisis" post-LM, this is likely to lessen as your body continues its recovery and becomes more adept at detoxification.

Tip:

With your surgeon's approval, incorporating anti-inflammatory supplements or detox teas into your regimen may help alleviate potential symptoms associated with a "detox crisis."

LEARN MORE:

Scan or click here to learn about ways to minimize a detox crisis after your LM.

54

WHAT IS EARLY INCISIONAL DRAINAGE MASSAGE?

Some surgeons advocate for post-surgical massage immediately following liposuction, aimed at minimizing fluid accumulation in tissues. In certain instances, the incisions at the liposuction cannula insertion points may be intentionally left open to allow fluid from the treated area to drain. These openings can remain patent, facilitating fluid drainage, for about twenty-four to forty-eight hours post-surgery.

During this initial twenty-four-to-forty-eight-hour period, massage therapists provide a specialized massage intended to expel as much fluid as possible through these openings, thus minimizing fluid retention in the liposuction areas. However, it's important to note that this type of massage is distinct from LM. It primarily focuses on forcing free fluid in the tissue to exit through the skin openings, rather than effectively removing fluid from the surgery site via the body's natural lymphatic pathways.

Note:

Early incision drainage massage can effectively expedite fluid removal, although it does come with certain challenges. A notable concern is that patients might experience a significant degree of pain and discomfort, as this technique is implemented just hours following the initial surgery. Moreover, logistical issues can add to the discomfort, with patients often facing considerable difficulties in transportation to the medical office on the first postoperative day.

Tip:

Before opting for early postoperative incisional massage, it's important to consult with your surgeon or LM therapist about whether this technique is typically utilized in their practice. You should have a detailed conversation about the benefits and potential drawbacks of this method, and perhaps inquire about the experiences of other patients who have previously undergone similar massage techniques. Making an informed decision based on this information will ensure you're well-prepared for what to expect.

LEARN MORE:

Scan or click here to learn more about pros and cons of incisional massage after liposuction.

55

WHAT IS DRAINING MASSAGE OR DRAIN MASSAGE?

"Drain massage" refers to a specific massage technique aimed at expelling free fluid from tissue by guiding it towards and into surgical drains that have been placed during a procedure. Surgeons often insert these drains into certain areas of the body to facilitate fluid removal, typically leaving them in place for several days to a few weeks.

When performing an LM, the therapist can take advantage of these existing drains. They can manipulate and guide free fluids towards these drains, enabling the fluid to exit the body. However, it's important to understand that while this massage technique can effectively reduce free fluid in the surgical area, it's distinct from traditional LM and should be seen as complementary to, rather than a replacement for, standard LM.

Once postoperative drains are removed, the emphasis shifts to traditional LM alone. This technique encourages the redirection of excessive body fluid from the surgical site through natural lymphatic pathways, assisting the body's inherent healing process.

Note:

It's worth noting that the practice of placing drains after circumferential body liposuction, also known as "360 Lipo," is quite common among plastic surgeons, predominantly in Latin America. This is done to facilitate the drainage of excessive fluid post-surgery. However, this technique is not broadly adopted in the United States. One potential drawback to consider is that these drains can become embedded in soft tissues, potentially causing pain or posing difficulties during postoperative removal.

Tip:

When preparing for surgery, including liposuction, it's advisable to ask your surgeon whether they plan on using drains during the procedure. Additionally, it's important to share this information with your LM specialist. Knowing if a drain will be used can help them tailor your postoperative LM protocol, ensuring that the treatment plan is as effective and comfortable for you as possible.

LEARN MORE:

Scan or click here to learn about benefits of drain massage.

56

CAN A LYMPHATIC MASSAGE THERAPIST REMOVE A DRAIN?

Typically, the removal of surgical drains is performed by a healthcare professional such as a doctor, nurse, or a specifically trained medical assistant. An LM therapist is not usually qualified or legally permitted to remove surgical drains, as this falls outside of their scope of practice. However, policies and regulations can vary by location and the specific certifications held by the therapist. It's crucial to always ensure any medical procedure is performed by a trained and authorized healthcare professional to guarantee safety and efficacy.

Note:

Removal of the drain should be performed by a trained healthcare provider and it requires technical skill and experience to troubleshoot potential problems with drain removal. Some potential complications may include:

1. **Pain or discomfort:** Some patients may experience pain or discomfort during or after the drain removal. However, this

is typically minimal and transient. 2. Infection: As with any surgical procedure, there's a risk of infection. Signs of infection may include redness, swelling, pain, or a fever.

2. **Seroma formation:** A seroma is a collection of fluid that builds up under the surface of your skin. It's one of the most common complications following drain removal after an abdominoplasty. If a seroma occurs, it may need to be drained by a healthcare professional.

3. **Hematoma:** This is a collection of blood outside of the blood vessels that may occur if a blood vessel is damaged during drain removal.

4. **Drain Retention:** There are instances when a portion of the drain is accidentally left inside. This could potentially lead to infection or cause a foreign body reaction.

5. **Delayed Healing:** Sometimes, the wound from the drain site may take longer to heal and could potentially lead to a noticeable scar.

6. **Numbness or altered sensation:** Some patients may experience changes in skin sensation around the drain site following removal. This is usually temporary.

Tip:

Always seek help from a healthcare professional for removal of a surgical drain.

LEARN MORE:

Scan or click here to learn about dangers of drain removal by a non-medical professional.

57

IS IT POSSIBLE TO RECEIVE A LYMPHATIC MASSAGE BEFORE THE DRAIN IS REMOVED?

Yes, LM can often be started even if a surgical drain is still in place after your surgery. In fact, LM can sometimes be beneficial in this context as it can help reduce fluid accumulation and swelling, which are the reasons the drain was placed to begin with.

However, it's important that the massage therapist is aware of the drain and works around it carefully to avoid causing any discomfort or dislodging the drain. Also, it's essential to choose a therapist who is experienced in working with post-surgical patients and be well-versed in the anatomy and physiology of the lymphatic system.

Note:

The structure of surgical drains is generally consistent. A surgical drain is a plastic tube with perforations at one end. Fluid is suctioned through these perforations located at the farthest end of the drain. To ensure effective drainage during an LM, the therapist must know the location of the drain's opposing end within the soft tissue. The position of the drains is determined during surgery. Although drains are most commonly placed around the incision site, their location can vary based on the surgeon's preferences.

Tip:

To maximize effectiveness of your LM and to minimize time with drains after surgery, ask your surgeon about the drain location and communicate this information to your LM therapist.

If you're keen on visualizing the extent of drainage facilitated during your massage session, it's advisable to empty out the accumulated blood and lymph fluid from the drains before your therapy begins. By doing so, post-session, you can clearly gauge the amount of fluid that has been mobilized and subsequently drained from your body through the drains. This practice not only provides a visual representation of the progress made but also may serve as a motivating factor in your recovery journey.

LEARN MORE:

Scan or click here to learn how to accurately measure drain output.

58

IS A DOCTOR'S ORDER OR PRESCRIPTION REQUIRED FOR LYMPHATIC MASSAGE?

The requirements for a doctor's order or prescription for LM can vary depending on your location, local regulations, insurance policies, and the specific practices of the massage therapist or clinic.

In many cases, a prescription may not be required. Many massage therapists can perform LM based on a patient's request. However, it is always a good idea to consult with your healthcare provider before starting any new treatment, including LM, especially after recovering from plastic surgery or if you have a specific medical condition.

If you are hoping to have the cost of the LM covered by your health insurance, you may need a doctor's prescription. Many insurance companies require a prescription to justify the medical necessity of the massage before they agree to cover the cost.

Note:

While LM is generally not covered by health insurance providers, coverage policies can vary between states. It is advisable to contact your health insurance company directly to inquire about the possibility of coverage for LM.

Tip:

Ask your LM beforehand if a doctor's order is required for sessions after surgery.

59

IS LYMPHATIC MASSAGE EFFECTIVE IF PERFORMED ONLY ONCE A WEEK?

The effectiveness of LM can vary based on several factors, including the frequency of sessions. While receiving LM once a week can still offer benefits, it may not yield the same optimal results as more frequent sessions.

If you are limited to receiving LM once a week, it is still worth pursuing as it can provide some benefits. However, for maximum effectiveness, it is generally recommended to follow the guidance of your healthcare provider or therapist regarding the frequency of LM sessions to best support your recovery.

Note:

Understanding the importance of the frequency of LM at different stages after surgery is crucial. To illustrate this, let's consider the analogy of a city experiencing a severe flood. When a flood suddenly hits the city, it paralyzes transportation and hinders essential functions. The city suffers from food and water shortages and first responders are unable to reach areas where help is needed. As the water gradually recedes, some essential city functions start to return, although not at full capacity. Transportation can resume, first responders can provide assistance, and essential services gradually return. Once all the water is removed, the city fully recovers, and all structures function well.

Similar processes can occur in the body after surgery, particularly following liposuction. After surgery, there is significant swelling (edema) as the tissues become overwhelmed with fluid and inflammatory molecules, hindering normal healing processes. LM plays a crucial role in removing excess fluid, restoring tissue function, and promoting proper healing. However, after each session of LM, the body slowly reabsorbs fluid back into the surgical sites, though in smaller volumes each time. This fluid accumulation hinders the body's ability to heal properly.

Therefore, periodic assistance with fluid removal through LM is necessary. The frequency of LM sessions may be higher in the early stages after surgery when fluid accumulation is significant, and then gradually decreases as the body's lymphatic system recovers and becomes more efficient in naturally removing fluid.

It's important to follow the guidance of your healthcare provider or therapist regarding the recommended frequency of LM sessions at different stages of your recovery. This will help optimize the benefits of LM and support your body's healing process.

Tip:

Discuss benefits of LM after surgery with your surgeon and massage therapist. LM continues to be beneficial at any stage of the healing process, providing ongoing support to the body's natural recovery mechanisms. One of the significant advantages of seeking the expertise of an experienced LM therapist is their ability to identify and address potential soft tissue healing issues that may have gone unnoticed. For instance, they can effectively address fibrosis, a condition where excess scar tissue forms in the affected area after surgery, which might otherwise have remained undiagnosed and untreated. By incorporating regular LM sessions into your wellness routine beyond the immediate recovery phase, you can proactively promote healthy lymphatic flow, reduce inflammation, and maintain optimal tissue health in the long run.

LEARN MORE:

Scan or click here to learn about recovery protocols after different plastic surgery procedures.

60

WHAT IS THE BASIC TECHNIQUE FOR LYMPHATIC MASSAGE AFTER 360 LIPOSUCTION?

Here is the basic technique for MLD that can be applied after a 360-liposuction procedure:

1. **Preparation:** The patient lies in a comfortable position, typically on a massage table. The therapist begins by activating the lymph nodes in various regions of the body, thereby enhancing the flow of lymphatic fluid within the circulatory system. This initial step is crucial before proceeding to further stimulate and eliminate excess fluid, effectively reducing edema.

2. **Light Pressure:** The therapist starts by applying gentle, rhythmic strokes using flat hands or fingertips on the skin. The pressure should be light and should not cause any discomfort.

3. **Sequential Movements:** The therapist uses specific sequences of movements to follow the natural pathways of

the lymphatic system. This typically involves gentle, stretching motions, circular motions, pumping or light massage strokes. The strokes are applied in one direction towards the closest lymph nodes, following the pathways of lymphatic watersheds, to facilitate lymphatic drainage.

4. **Progression:** The therapist gradually moves from one area to another, working systematically around the body. For a 360-liposuction procedure, the therapist may start with the upper body, moving from the neck, shoulders, and arms towards the axillary lymph nodes. Then, they may move to the lower body, focusing on the abdomen, hips, buttocks, and legs, directing the strokes towards the inguinal lymph nodes. Your massage therapist might suggest various body positions during the session, tailored to the specific areas being treated. For instance, releasing fibrotic tissue in the flanks may be most effective with you in a side-lying position. For massaging areas treated by liposuction, such as the back, a face-down or side-lying position might be employed. The choice of position will depend on both the type of surgery you've undergone and your stage of recovery, ensuring the process is both safe and comfortable for you.

5. **Light Pressure around Incisions:** If the incisions from the liposuction procedure are healed and cleared by the surgeon, the therapist may gently apply light pressure around the incision sites to facilitate fluid movement and minimize scar tissue formation. However, this should be done with caution and only if approved by the surgeon. Once scar tissue is fully healed, typically by weeks six to eight, with all tissue structures closed, a trained therapist can incorporate various massage tools to prevent adhesion build-ups and address irregular or hardened tissues. Techniques include manual methods like counter-friction and deeper tissue maneuvers,

as well as tools like cupping therapy and gua sha. While most techniques aim to increase heat and circulation, thereby flattening the tissue, cupping therapy uniquely lifts and separates tissue layers, enhancing blood flow and toxin removal. However, caution is essential with cupping in post-operative care to ensure complete wound healing and the absence of soreness or bruising. Its usage may be intense or mildly uncomfortable but is highly effective for breaking up scar tissue, fibrotic tissue, and tight muscle bands. Continuous communication between the therapist and client is key to maintaining a relaxed and comfortable massage session.

Note:

LM techniques can vary among therapists, influenced by their training, level of knowledge, and personal experience. However, it is important that any variation in LM technique incorporates the basic principles outlined in the classic teachings of Dr. Vodder.

Dr. Vodder is renowned for his contributions to the field of MLD. His teachings emphasize the specific sequences and gentle, rhythmic movements that are characteristic of MLD. These techniques are designed to stimulate the lymphatic system, promote lymph flow, and encourage the removal of waste products and excess fluid from the body. During your massage session, various methods and tools may be utilized, depending on the massage therapist's advanced training. Therapists working in post-operative care often pursue additional education in techniques like wood therapy, cupping therapy, kinesio taping, and cavitation therapy, each offering unique benefits for body contouring and reducing swelling. It's advisable to inquire about your therapist's qualifications in these areas. While some may have learned from online sources, professional therapists typically display certifications or licenses in their offices as proof of their formal training and expertise in these specialized therapies.

While therapists may bring their unique style and approach to MLD, adhering to the fundamental principles outlined by Dr. Vodder ensures a solid foundation for effective and safe treatment. These principles include the use of light pressure, following the natural pathways of the lymphatic system, and considering the individual needs and condition of each client.

By incorporating these basic principles, therapists can provide a consistent and reliable standard of care, while still allowing for the necessary adaptations and modifications based on individual circumstances.

Tip:

It is always beneficial to seek out therapists who have received proper training and are knowledgeable in the principles and techniques of MLD to ensure a high-quality and effective treatment experience.

Strict compression and regular lymphatic massage (LM) are crucial following 360 lipo, as it involves liposuction over a large area of the body. The use of back compression devices, like a lumbar board, can be particularly beneficial in this context.

 **LEARN MORE:** Scan or click here to learn about surgical techniques and the recovery process after 360 lipo.

61

WHAT IS THE BASIC TECHNIQUE FOR LYMPHATIC MASSAGE AFTER BBL?

LM can be beneficial after a Brazilian butt lift (BBL) to help reduce swelling, promote healing, and optimize the results. Here is the basic technique for MLD that can be applied during LM after a BBL:

The therapist begins by activating the lymph nodes in various regions of the body, thereby enhancing the flow of lymphatic fluid within the circulatory system. This initial step is crucial before proceeding to further stimulate and eliminate excess fluid, effectively reducing edema.

1. **Preparation:** The patient is positioned comfortably, either standing in front of a massage table draped in a bathrobe, or seated upright on the table with a BBL pillow under their hamstrings. Some therapists may prefer having the client kneel on the massage table. All these positions are suitable as long as the patient avoids sitting directly on any area that has recently undergone fat grafting to the buttocks. Applying

pressure to this area can harm the newly grafted fat cells, which is why plastic surgeons advise their clients on how long they should avoid sitting post-surgery. Both patient and therapist work together to create a calm and relaxed environment for the session.

2. **Gentle Strokes:** The therapist begins by applying very gentle, light strokes on the skin surrounding the buttocks and the areas where liposuction was performed. The pressure should be soft and soothing.

3. **Sequential Movements:** Using specific sequences of movements, the therapist follows the natural pathways of the lymphatic system. These movements may include gentle stretching motions, circular motions, pumping actions, or light massage strokes. The strokes are directed towards the nearest lymph nodes to encourage lymphatic drainage.

4. **Focused Areas:** The therapist pays particular attention to the areas where liposuction was performed, such as the lower back, waist, and hips. They may use gentle, targeted techniques to help reduce swelling and promote fluid movement in these specific areas.

5. **Abdominal Massage:** If the abdomen was also involved in the BBL procedure, the therapist may incorporate gentle abdominal massage techniques to aid in lymphatic drainage and support overall healing.

6. **Education and Self-Care:** The therapist may also provide education on self-care techniques, such as proper positioning, breathing exercises, and gentle movements that can be done at home to further support lymphatic drainage.

Note:

BBL is a procedure that involves a combination of traditional body liposuction, typically 360-lipo, and the injection of harvested and processed fat into the buttock area. In terms of postoperative LM therapy, the liposuction areas are treated similarly to any other liposuctioned areas with LM techniques. However, it's important to note that applying significant pressure to the buttock area, where fat injections were performed, is contraindicated for a period of two to eight weeks following surgery.

Many surgeons advise against massaging the buttock area during this time frame. This precaution is taken to protect the newly injected fat cells and ensure their optimal survival and integration into the buttock tissues. Applying pressure or manipulating the area can potentially disrupt the healing process and compromise the desired outcome.

It is crucial to follow your surgeon's specific postoperative instructions and guidelines regarding LM and the care of the buttock area after a BBL. By adhering to these recommendations, you can promote optimal healing, minimize the risk of complications, and achieve the best possible results from your BBL procedure.

Tip:

Prior to undergoing surgery, it is important to have a discussion with your surgeon regarding the postoperative LM techniques that can be applied over the buttock area following fat injection, as well as the appropriate timing for such treatments.

By consulting your surgeon, you can gain a clear understanding of their specific recommendations and guidelines. They will provide insights into when it is safe to proceed with LM in the buttock region after the fat injection procedure. This information is crucial to ensure the optimal healing and integration of the injected fat cells, while minimizing the risk of complications.

Each surgeon may have their own approach and postoperative protocols, so it is essential to Have a conversation directly with your surgeon to address any concerns or questions you may have. This communication will enable you to make informed decisions and follow the appropriate postoperative care plan, resulting in the best possible outcomes from your surgery.

LEARN MORE:

Scan or click here for more information about the BBL surgical technique.

62

WHAT IS THE BASIC TECHNIQUE FOR MANUAL LYMPHATIC DRAINAGE AFTER A TUMMY TUCK?

The lymphatic drainage technique used after abdominoplasty differs from post liposuction lymphatic drainage, primarily due to the direction of the strokes. The therapist begins by activating the lymph nodes in various regions of the body, thereby enhancing the flow of lymphatic fluid within the circulatory system. This initial step is crucial before proceeding to further stimulate and eliminate excess fluid, effectively reducing edema.

Following liposuction, the strokes are directed from the center of the anterior abdomen (umbilical area) towards the main lymphatic flow regional collectors, such as the groin, to facilitate fluid outflow through the body's natural lymphatic tract. Although the lymphatic structures may be impacted by surgical trauma, they generally remain intact after the procedure.

However, abdominoplasty involves a wide transverse low abdominal incision that completely severs all lymphatic pathways from the abdomen to the groin. Additionally, dissection over the muscle and separation of the superior abdominal flap disrupt lymphatic outflow from the area.

As lymphatic flow through the incision is not possible, LM aims to redirect fluid into alternative regional lymph collectors (e.g., from the lower abdominal area to the armpit nodes) by activating remaining lymphatic collaterals. Therefore, the strokes above abdominal incision should be directed sideways and superiorly towards the underarm lymph nodes, while strokes below the incision should be directed towards the right and left groin areas.

It is crucial to emphasize that there are situations where LM therapists may need to use strokes over the stomach towards the incision. This maneuver could be necessary to move free subcutaneous fluid towards the drain area when a surgical drain is present.

However, it's important to note that such strokes will push fluid with soft tissue towards the transected lymphatic pathway, thereby failing to eliminate fluid in this area via the natural lymphatic pathways. While this technique may be used temporarily to facilitate fluid movement towards the drain, it should be done with caution and only as long as the surgical drain is in place.

Once the drain is removed, it becomes essential to avoid strokes towards the incision and instead focus on redirecting fluid towards alternative regional lymph collectors, as discussed previously. This approach ensures that the lymphatic system is supported in draining excess fluid effectively and promotes proper healing and recovery after abdominoplasty.

Note:

Unfortunately, not all LM providers are aware of this crucial concept. Some therapists, especially those without specific training, may unknowingly attempt to perform strokes in the wrong direction after abdominoplasty.

Tip:

Due to the presence of a lower abdominal incision, the most significant postoperative challenge for the lymphatic and vascular systems is located below the umbilicus. The triangle area extending from the umbilicus down to the corners of the abdominal incision (referred to as the "swollen triangle" area) is notorious for delayed healing and prolonged residual edema, even with massage and compression. However, the good news is that over time, the edema in this area gradually subsides as well.

LEARN MORE:

Scan or click here to learn more about the abdominoplasty surgical technique and recovery process.

63

IS LYMPHATIC MASSAGE AFTER 360 LIPOSUCTION DIFFERENT FROM POST BBL MASSAGE?

When discussing postoperative care, particularly LM, it's important to understand that different surgical procedures, such as 360 liposuction and BBL, require tailored approaches. In 360 liposuction, fat is removed from the entire circumference of the midsection, including the abdomen, flanks, back, and sometimes thighs. The LM post-360 liposuction focuses on this large area, helping to reduce swelling and prevent fluid accumulation, thereby enhancing circulation and facilitating healing. Patients are required to wear comprehensive compression garments to ensure even pressure and support for the entire treated area.

On the other hand, BBL, a two-step process involving liposuction and fat transfer to the buttocks, demands a more delicate approach in lymphatic massage, especially around the buttocks. The aim here is to promote healing and reduce swelling in the liposuction areas while avoiding direct pressure on the buttocks to protect the newly grafted fat cells. Post-BBL patients must avoid sitting directly on their buttocks for a certain period, and the LMs are meticulously performed to avoid pressure on the fat grafting area. The compression garments used are specifically designed to compress the liposuction areas without putting pressure on the buttocks.

The key differences in the postoperative LM between these two procedures lie in the area of massage focus, application of pressure, and the goals of the massage. In 360 lipo, the massage covers a more extensive area, whereas in BBL, the emphasis is more on liposuction sites, with special precautions to avoid the buttocks. While both procedures use LM to reduce swelling and improve healing, BBL massages also aim to protect the fat transfer to the buttocks.

Understanding these nuances is crucial for patients undergoing either procedure, ensuring they receive the appropriate postoperative care, especially in terms of lymphatic massage. It's vital to consult with a healthcare provider or trained massage therapist for personalized care post-surgery for optimal results and a smooth recovery.

Note:

It's essential to emphasize that the technique may vary depending on the therapist's training and the specific needs of the patient. The therapist should always adapt the treatment to suit individual circumstances while adhering to the basic principles of MLD.

Tip:

Strict compression and regular LM are crucial following either procedure, as both involve liposuction over a large area of the body. The use of back compression devices, like a lumbar board, can be particularly beneficial in this context.

 **LEARN MORE:** Scan or click <u>here</u> to learn about surgical technique and the recovery process after 360 lipo.

64

WHAT ESSENTIAL RECOVERY EQUIPMENT CAN HELP POST BBL RECOVERY?

Undergoing BBL is a transformative journey, and recovery plays a pivotal role in achieving the desired results. To ensure a smooth and successful healing process, it's important to have the right equipment on hand. This information will guide you through the essential items needed for recovery after a BBL, highlighting the importance of compression garments, BBL pillows, and other recovery aids.

A must-have after a BBL, compression garments are designed to support the areas treated during liposuction. They help reduce swelling, provide support to the surgical areas, and aid in the body contouring process. It's crucial to choose a garment that fits well— it should be snug but not excessively tight. Your surgeon will typically recommend how long to wear it for optimal results.

A BBL pillow is specially designed to protect and support your newly transferred fat cells when sitting. It allows you to sit without putting direct pressure on your buttocks, thus preserving the shape and viability of the fat grafts. This pillow will be your constant companion in the weeks following surgery, especially when sitting in a car or on a chair.

Since sleeping directly on your back or buttocks is off-limits after a BBL, you'll need to adjust your sleeping position. Special pillows can help you comfortably sleep on your stomach or side. Investing in a few extra pillows to support your legs and abdomen can also make sleeping in these new positions more comfortable.

Foam pads can be used in conjunction with your compression garment to provide additional support and contouring to specific areas, like the abdomen or back. These pads can help prevent fluid accumulation and aid in smoother recovery.

Your skin will need extra care as it heals. Gentle, hydrating lotions and scar treatment creams can be beneficial, especially on areas where liposuction was performed. Always check with your surgeon before applying anything to your incisions.

For managing pain and swelling, have some ice packs ready. You can also use heating pads to ease muscle soreness in areas like the back, which might be strained due to altered sleeping positions.

Stock your closet with loose, comfortable clothing that's easy to put on and take off. Clothing that doesn't press against your treatment areas is ideal, especially in the first few weeks post-surgery.

Note:

It is extremely important to avoid direct pressure over fat grafted buttocks during the postoperative period. To avoid pressure over the buttocks after a Brazilian Butt Lift (BBL) and ensure a successful recovery, consider the following tips:

1. Use specialized cushions: Invest in a BBL pillow or cushion designed to relieve pressure on the buttocks. These cushions

have a cutout in the center, allowing you to sit without putting direct pressure on the newly transferred fat.

2. Follow postoperative instructions: Strictly adhere to your plastic surgeon's postoperative guidelines. These may include avoiding sitting or lying directly on your buttocks for a specific period after surgery.

3. Opt for alternative seating positions: During the initial recovery phase, try sitting on your thighs or using a kneeling chair. This way, you can keep pressure off the buttocks while providing support to other parts of your body.

4. Change positions regularly: If you must sit, make an effort to shift your weight and change positions frequently. Avoid sitting in one position for an extended period to reduce pressure on the buttocks.

5. Lay on your side: When resting or sleeping, lie on your side rather than on your back or buttocks to alleviate pressure.

6. Avoid driving long distances: Refrain from driving long distances for a few weeks post-surgery to minimize pressure on the buttocks while sitting.

7. Use proper technique for standing and sitting: When standing up from a seated position, do so with care to avoid putting excessive pressure on the buttocks.

8. Wear loose-fitting clothing: Choose clothing that doesn't compress the buttocks, as tight garments may impede proper blood circulation and put additional pressure on the area.

9. Stay hydrated and nourished: Proper hydration and nutrition play a vital role in supporting the healing process and promoting better blood flow.

10. Communicate with your surgeon: If you have any concerns or questions about avoiding pressure on the buttocks during recovery, don't hesitate to communicate with your plastic surgeon. They can provide personalized advice to ensure a smooth and successful healing process.

Tip:

A portable female urinal is an indispensable tool for recovery after a Brazilian Butt Lift (BBL). Following this procedure, it's crucial to limit pressure on the buttocks to ensure the best possible healing and fat graft survival. This restriction can make regular bathroom visits challenging, as traditional sitting positions are not advisable.

The portable female urinal offers a practical solution to this issue. It allows for easy urination while standing or in a semi-upright position, effectively reducing the need to sit and thus minimizing pressure on the sensitive areas. This can be particularly helpful during the initial weeks post-surgery when the healing process is most critical, and maintaining the shape and integrity of the buttock augmentation is paramount.

Furthermore, the convenience of a portable urinal cannot be overstated, especially for those who might have difficulty moving around immediately after surgery. It adds an element of independence to personal care and hygiene during recovery, which can be both empowering and comforting for patients. Additionally, it helps maintain a level of dignity and ease during a time that can often be challenging and uncomfortable.

Incorporating a portable female urinal into your post-BBL recovery plan can significantly enhance your comfort and contribute to a smoother, more manageable healing journey. It's a small investment that can make a significant difference in the overall recovery experience. As always, it's important to follow your surgeon's specific postoperative care instructions and to discuss any concerns or additional needs you might have during your recovery.

 **LEARN MORE:** Scan or click here to learn about the top ten must have recovery items after BBL.

65

WHEN CAN LYMPHATIC MASSAGE OF THE BUTTOCKS BE STARTED AFTER A BBL PROCEDURE?

The timing for starting buttock massage after a BBL surgery can vary depending on individual factors and the surgeon's postoperative instructions. Generally, it is crucial to follow your surgeon's specific guidelines and recommendations, as they are familiar with the details of your procedure and can provide personalized advice.

In most cases, massage of the buttock area, where the fat grafts were injected, is typically avoided during the early stages of recovery. The first few weeks after surgery are critical for the newly transferred fat cells to establish blood supply and integrate into the surrounding tissues. Applying pressure or manipulating the area too soon could potentially disrupt the healing process and affect the final results.

Surgeons may advise patients to avoid any direct pressure on the buttock area for a certain period, usually ranging from two to eight weeks. During this time, it's essential to focus on other areas that have undergone liposuction, using manual lymphatic drainage techniques to reduce swelling and promote healing.

Note:

Always communicate with your surgeon and seek their guidance on when you can start massaging the buttock area safely. Following their instructions will help ensure a smooth recovery and optimize the long-term results of your BBL surgery. To maintain the best outcome and ensure the longevity of the fat graft, it is essential to follow your plastic surgeon's specific postoperative instructions regarding sitting, lying, and avoiding pressure on the buttocks. In some cases, surgeons may recommend using specialized cushions or pillows that relieve pressure on the buttocks while sitting.

TipS:

1. **Use a BBL Pillow for Sitting:** When you need to sit, use a specially designed BBL pillow. These pillows allow you to sit without putting direct pressure on your buttocks by supporting your thighs and elevating your rear off the surface. This is crucial for maintaining the integrity of the newly transferred fat cells.

2. **Adopt the Right Sleeping Position:** Sleeping on your stomach is ideal post-BBL to avoid pressure on the buttocks. If you can't sleep on your stomach, try sleeping on your side with the help of body pillows for support. Avoid sleeping on your back until your surgeon gives you the go-ahead.

3. **Knee Position for Meal Times:** When eating, consider kneeling on a pillow or soft surface with your buttocks lifted off your heels. You can use a yoga mat for additional cushioning. This position relieves pressure on the buttocks while allowing you to sit upright at a table.

4. **Avoid Driving:** Driving should be avoided for the first few weeks after surgery, as sitting in a car seat can put pressure on the buttocks. If you must travel by car, use a BBL pillow and try to limit the time spent in the car as much as possible.

5. **Limit Sitting Time:** Even with a BBL pillow, it's important to limit the total time spent sitting. Aim to stand or lie down every thirty minutes to ensure there isn't constant pressure on the buttocks.

6. **Gentle Walking:** Short, gentle walks can help improve circulation and reduce the risk of blood clots. Walking also allows you to be upright and off your buttocks, giving the area time to heal.

7. **Adjustable Bed or Recliner Chair:** If available, use an adjustable bed or a recliner chair for relaxation. These can be set to a position that takes pressure off the buttocks while still allowing you to be somewhat upright.

8. **Use a Mattress Topper:** For additional comfort while sleeping, consider adding a soft mattress topper. This can provide extra cushioning and help distribute your weight more evenly when lying down.

9. **Follow Surgeon's Guidelines:** Always follow the specific postoperative instructions provided by your surgeon. They might have additional advice based on the specifics of your surgery and individual healing process.

10. **Stay Patient and Follow Up:** Recovery from a BBL takes time, and it's important to be patient and stick to these guidelines for the recommended period. Also, make sure to attend all follow-up appointments with your surgeon to monitor your healing progress.

LEARN MORE: Scan or click <u>here</u> to learn more about healing of the grafted buttock fat after BBL.

66

WHAT IS THE BASIC TECHNIQUE FOR MANUAL LYMPHATIC DRAINAGE AFTER BREAST REDUCTION OR LIFT?

The basic technique for LM after breast reduction or lift involves gentle, rhythmic movements to support the lymphatic system and promote fluid drainage. Here is a simple outline of the technique:

1. **Preparation:** The patient lies comfortably on a massage table, ensuring a relaxed and comfortable position. The therapist begins by activating the lymph nodes in various regions of the body, thereby enhancing the flow of lymphatic fluid within the circulatory system. This initial step is crucial before proceeding to further stimulate and eliminate excess fluid, effectively reducing edema.

2. **Gentle Strokes:** The therapist starts with very light, gentle strokes on the skin surrounding the breasts, focusing on the chest, underarms, and upper torso. These strokes are applied

with soft pressure to avoid any discomfort or strain on the surgical area.

3. **Sequential Movements:** Using specific sequences of movements, the therapist follows the natural pathways of the lymphatic system. These may include gentle stretching motions, circular motions, or pumping actions, all designed to encourage lymph flow and fluid movement.

4. **Drainage of Lymph Nodes:** Special attention is given to the lymph nodes in the underarm area (axillary nodes) and around the breasts. The therapist may use techniques to stimulate fluid drainage towards these regional lymph collectors.

5. **Avoiding Pressure on Incisions:** It is essential for the therapist to avoid applying direct pressure on the incision sites where the breast reduction or lift surgery was performed. The goal is to support fluid drainage without disturbing the healing process.

6. **Post-Treatment Care:** After the session, the therapist may provide instructions for self-care techniques, such as gentle arm movements and deep breathing exercises, to further support lymphatic drainage between sessions.

Note:

It's important to note that the technique may vary depending on the therapist's training and the specific needs of the patient. The therapist should always adapt the treatment to suit individual circumstances while adhering to the basic principles of MLD.

Tip:

The type of LM techniques used after breast reduction or breast lift surgery should always be coordinated with the surgeon. Both procedures can be performed using distinct surgical techniques that may disrupt the natural lymphatic pathways in unique ways. As a result, post-surgical massage techniques need to be tailored to the specific surgical method of reduction or lift and must be adapted depending on the degree of post-surgical anatomy changes.

When seeking an LM therapist after breast surgery, it's essential to inquire about their experience and expertise with clients who have undergone breast procedures. A specialist should have a clear understanding of the differences between techniques used in various breast surgeries. For instance, LM techniques applied after breast cancer surgery can differ significantly from those used after cosmetic breast procedures. Therefore, look for an LM therapist with specific experience in post-cosmetic breast procedures to ensure the best possible care.

By choosing a qualified and knowledgeable LM therapist who understands the unique aspects of breast surgery and its impact on the lymphatic system, you can receive tailored and effective MLD results that support your healing and recovery process. Coordinating with your surgeon and finding the right LM specialist will contribute to the successful outcome of your breast reduction or lift surgery.

LEARN MORE:

Scan or click here to learn more about the benefits of LM after breast reduction.

67

WHAT IS THE BASIC TECHNIQUE FOR MANUAL LYMPHATIC DRAINAGE AFTER BREAST IMPLANT SURGERY?

The basic technique for manual lymphatic drainage (MLD) after breast implant surgery involves gentle, rhythmic movements to promote fluid drainage and support the lymphatic system. Here is a simple outline of the technique:

1. **Preparation:** The patient lies comfortably on a massage table, ensuring a relaxed and comfortable position. The therapist begins by activating the lymph nodes in various regions of the body, thereby enhancing the flow of lymphatic fluid within the circulatory system. This initial step is crucial before proceeding to further stimulate and eliminate excess fluid, effectively reducing edema.

2. **Gentle Strokes:** The therapist starts with very light, gentle strokes on the skin surrounding the breasts, focusing on the chest, underarms, and upper torso. These strokes are applied

with soft pressure to avoid any discomfort or strain on the surgical area.

3. **Sequential Movements:** Using specific sequences of movements, the therapist follows the natural pathways of the lymphatic system. These may include gentle stretching motions, circular motions, or pumping actions, all designed to encourage lymph flow and fluid movement.

4. **Focus on Drainage Areas:** Special attention is given to the lymph nodes in the underarm area (axillary nodes) and around the breasts. The therapist may use techniques to stimulate fluid drainage towards these regional lymph collectors.

5. **Avoiding Pressure on Implants:** It is essential for the therapist to avoid applying direct pressure on the breast implants or incision sites. The goal is to support fluid drainage without disturbing the healing process or affecting the implants.

6. **Post-Treatment Care:** After the session, the therapist may provide instructions for self-care techniques, such as gentle arm movements and deep breathing exercises, to further support lymphatic drainage between sessions.

Note:

Most surgeons recommend avoiding any manipulation of the breasts after breast augmentation with implants. Typically, after this surgery, it is essential to provide good support for the breasts and stabilize them until the natural support system for the implants has developed, which usually takes about six to eight weeks. As a result, LM may not be recommended by surgeons for several weeks after the procedure.

Always follow your surgeon's instructions, as they possess the best knowledge of the surgical anatomy and the specifics of your surgery. Various intra-operative factors, such as the position of the implant, volume, and quality of the tissue, can be reasons for the surgeon to further delay LM after breast augmentation.

It's important to prioritize your healing and recovery, and adhering to your surgeon's recommendations is vital. As your body adjusts to the implants and the surgical site heals, the timing for introducing LM can vary. Trust in your surgeon's expertise and communicate openly with them about any concerns or questions you may have regarding postoperative care.

Tip:

Having breast augmentation, with or without a lift, in combination with other body cosmetic surgical procedures, such as abdominoplasty or body liposuction, does not preclude the performance of MLD for other body areas.

In fact, integrating MLD into your postoperative care regimen can offer numerous benefits for your overall recovery. While the surgical focus may be on specific areas, the body's lymphatic system is interconnected, and MLD can positively impact the entire body's fluid balance and immune function.

For instance, after breast augmentation surgery, MLD can help reduce swelling, promote the healing process, and enhance lymphatic circulation in the chest, shoulders, and arms. Similarly, following procedures like abdominoplasty or liposuction, MLD can aid in reducing swelling in the abdominal region and other treated areas, such as the hips and thighs.

By considering MLD for the appropriate areas, you can optimize the healing process, alleviate discomfort, and enhance the overall surgical outcome. It's essential to work with a qualified and experienced LM therapist who understands your unique surgical procedures and can provide specialized care to support your recovery journey effectively.

Remember to discuss incorporating MLD into your postoperative care plan with both your surgeon and LM therapist. Their collaborative approach will ensure that your recovery is well-coordinated, safe, and tailored to your specific needs.

LEARN MORE:

Scan or click here to find out more about the benefits of LM for recovery after breast augmentation.

68

WHAT IS THE BASIC TECHNIQUE FOR MANUAL LYMPHATIC DRAINAGE AFTER AN ARM LIPOSUCTION OR LIFT?

The basic technique for MLD after an arm liposuction or lift involves gentle, rhythmic movements to promote fluid drainage and support the lymphatic system. Here is a simple outline of the technique:

1. **Preparation:** The patient lies comfortably on a massage table, ensuring a relaxed and comfortable position. The therapist begins by activating the lymph nodes in various regions of the body, thereby enhancing the flow of lymphatic fluid within the circulatory system. This initial step is crucial before proceeding to further stimulate and eliminate excess fluid, effectively reducing edema.

2. **Gentle Strokes:** The therapist starts with very light, gentle strokes on the skin surrounding the arms, including the upper arms and underarms. These strokes are applied with soft

pressure to avoid any discomfort or strain on the surgical areas.

3. **Sequential Movements:** Using specific sequences of movements, the therapist follows the natural pathways of the lymphatic system in the arms. These may include gentle stretching motions, circular motions, or pumping actions, all designed to encourage lymph flow and fluid movement.

4. **Focus on Drainage Areas:** Special attention is given to the lymph nodes in the underarm area (axillary nodes) and around the elbows. The therapist may use techniques to stimulate fluid drainage towards these regional lymph collectors.

5. **Avoiding Pressure on Incisions:** It is essential for the therapist to avoid applying direct pressure on the incision sites or areas where liposuction was performed. The goal is to support fluid drainage without disturbing the healing process.

6. **Post-Treatment Care:** After the session, the therapist may provide instructions for self-care techniques, such as gentle arm movements and deep breathing exercises, to further support lymphatic drainage between sessions.

Note:

The basic technique for MLD after upper arm liposuction or arm lift involves gentle, rhythmic movements to promote fluid drainage and support the lymphatic system. However, some differences in MLD techniques may be seen based on the specific surgical procedures used.

After upper arm liposuction, MLD focuses on promoting lymphatic drainage by applying strokes circumferentially around the arms. This helps to encourage the movement of fluid and reduce swelling in the treated areas.

In contrast, after an arm lift, special care and precaution are taken when treating areas with surgical incisions in the inner arms. The therapist will apply gentle strokes to these areas to support the healing process and minimize any potential discomfort.

Overall, the main goal of MLD after both liposuction and arm lift procedures is to reduce swelling, promote healing, and optimize the overall recovery process. The techniques used may vary slightly based on the surgical approach, but the underlying principles of MLD remain consistent.

Liposuction performed on the arms can often result in the development of fibrotic tissue, leading to symptoms such as bruising, warmth, and heightened sensitivity. After the surgical procedure, patients typically experience limited mobility in their arms. It is crucial to prioritize the comfort of the client during massage sessions in these cases. To facilitate the movement of fluids towards the axillary lymph nodes, a therapist may gently position the client's arm or support it with a pillow.

Initially, it is advisable to apply very gentle pressure during the massage, employing standard MLD techniques with a delicate fingertip touch. Pain-relief creams can be utilized to alleviate any discomfort that may arise during the early sessions. Although post-operative swelling is common, fibrosis in the arm can be more persistent. As the massage sessions progress, the therapist may gradually increase the pressure to assist in the removal of fluids and the breakdown of fibrotic tissue.

Self-massage and the use of arm compression garments are indispensable for achieving optimal recovery. With guidance from a trained therapist, patients can cautiously work towards regaining their full range of motion in the arms over time.

To ensure the best results and safe recovery, it is essential to work with a qualified and experienced LM therapist who understands the nuances of post-upper arm surgical care. They can provide tailored MLD techniques to support your healing journey effectively and achieve the desired outcomes of your surgical procedure.

Tip:

Utilize the power of gravity to facilitate the functioning of the arm lymphatic system. Frequent and prolonged elevation of the arms can have a significant positive impact on fluid transition from surgical sites to the axillary lymphatic collectors. Elevating the arms above heart level encourages the natural flow of lymph, aiding in the reduction of swelling and promoting a faster recovery process after arm lift or liposuction procedures.

To complement arm elevation, consider wearing a comfortable and effective arm compression garment. Compression garments provide gentle pressure on the treated areas, helping to support the lymphatic system and further minimize swelling. The combination of arm elevation and compression promotes better fluid drainage, reducing the accumulation of excess fluid and expediting the healing process.

Additionally, practicing deep breathing exercises can aid in enhancing lymphatic circulation, as the movement of the diaphragm helps to stimulate the lymphatic vessels and encourage fluid flow.

LEARN MORE:

Scan or click here to learn more tips for recovering from arm lift surgery.

69

What is the Basic Technique for Manual Lymphatic Drainage after Thigh Liposuction or Lift?

The basic technique for manual lymphatic drainage (MLD) after thigh liposuction or lift involves gentle, rhythmic movements to promote fluid drainage and support the lymphatic system. Here is a simple outline of the technique:

1. **Preparation:** The patient lies comfortably on a massage table, ensuring a relaxed and comfortable position. For thigh liposuction, the therapist will focus on the treated areas, while for thigh lift, the entire thigh region will be considered. The therapist begins by activating the lymph nodes in various regions of the body, thereby enhancing the flow of lymphatic fluid within the circulatory system. This initial step is crucial before proceeding to further stimulate and eliminate excess fluid, effectively reducing edema.

2. **Gentle Strokes:** The therapist starts with very light, gentle strokes on the skin surrounding the thighs, including the front, back, inner, and outer areas. These strokes are applied with soft pressure to avoid any discomfort or strain on the surgical areas.

3. **Sequential Movements:** Using specific sequences of movements, the therapist follows the natural pathways of the lymphatic system in the thighs. These may include gentle stretching motions, circular motions, or pumping actions, all designed to encourage lymph flow and fluid movement. When focusing on the inner thighs during a massage, it's beneficial to position the client in a "figure four" arrangement. In this position, the leg is oriented so that the knee faces the side of the table, and the bottom of the foot may come into contact with the opposite leg. This positioning allows the therapist to have unobstructed access to the inner thigh area. The therapist should use gentle strokes, massaging from the knee towards the inguinal lymph nodes.

Following inner thigh surgery, the region can be highly sensitive during the initial one to three sessions. Effective communication between the therapist and the patient is essential to monitor and address any discomfort. The primary objective is to reduce swelling and address the presence of fibrotic or uneven tissue. As you progress from weeks three to five, consider incorporating light deep tissue massage techniques, cupping therapy, and wood therapy to help break down unwanted fibrotic tissue in the legs, further enhancing body contouring.

For the lateral thigh area, it is advisable for the therapist to position the client on their side during the massage. This positioning fully exposes the entire leg, ensuring a more effective massage session and achieving better outcomes. The application of pain-relief creams to the legs may also provide some relief.

If swelling extends to the lower leg and extremities, the therapist should massage the entire leg and recommend that the client wear compression garments for a minimum of two weeks. This comprehensive approach contributes to a smoother and more comfortable recovery process.

4. **Focus on Drainage Areas:** Special attention is given to the lymph nodes in the groin and inner thigh areas. The therapist may use techniques to stimulate fluid drainage towards these regional lymph collectors.

5. **Avoiding Pressure on Incisions:** It is essential for the therapist to avoid applying direct pressure on the incision sites or areas where liposuction was performed. The goal is to support fluid drainage without disturbing the healing process.

6. **Post-Treatment Care** After the session, the therapist may provide instructions for self-care techniques, such as gentle leg movements and deep breathing exercises, to further support lymphatic drainage between sessions.

Note:

One of the primary challenges during the recovery from thigh cosmetic surgeries, such as thigh lift, liposuction, or a combination of both, is the management of edema fluid. This fluid needs to be effectively drained out from the treated areas, moving from bottom up, against the force of gravity. Unlike the venous system, which efficiently pushes fluid towards the heart, the lymphatic system has a more challenging task in transporting fluid against gravity.

As a result, it becomes even more crucial for the LM (LM) therapist to play a significant role in facilitating fluid transit from the thighs after such surgeries. With skillful MLD techniques, the therapist can support the lymphatic system in its efforts to remove excess fluid, reduce swelling, and promote a smoother recovery.

The LM therapist employs gentle, rhythmic strokes and sequences that follow the natural pathways of the lymphatic system. Special attention is given to the groin area and surrounding lymph nodes, which are essential for the drainage of the thighs. By stimulating fluid movement and encouraging lymph flow, the therapist helps the body's natural drainage process, assisting in the reduction of postoperative edema.

Additionally, the therapist may recommend specific self-care techniques to complement the MLD sessions. These may include gentle leg exercises, deep breathing, and maintaining proper hydration, which all contribute to supporting the lymphatic system and optimizing fluid transit.

Tip:

The power of leg elevation lies in its ability to harness gravity to assist the lymphatic system in draining excess fluid from the lower extremities. When the legs are elevated, fluid is encouraged to flow in the right direction, moving from the ankles and calves upwards towards the thighs and groin. This reduces the pooling of fluid in the lower limbs, alleviating swelling and promoting a more efficient fluid transit process.

To optimize the benefits of leg elevation, try to maintain this position regularly throughout the day, especially during periods of rest and relaxation. While lying in bed or sitting, prop your legs up with pillows or cushions to ensure proper elevation. When seated, keep your feet elevated on a footrest or ottoman to maintain the desired position.

Furthermore, wearing compression garments on the lower extremities offers additional support in managing edema. Compression garments apply gentle pressure, aiding in fluid movement and reducing the risk of excessive swelling.

LEARN MORE:

Scan or click here to learn more recovery tips for after thigh liposuction.

$\underline{70}$

WHAT IS THE BASIC TECHNIQUE FOR MANUAL LYMPHATIC DRAINAGE AFTER A FACE LIFT?

The basic technique for MLD after a face lift involves gentle, precise movements to promote lymphatic flow and reduce swelling in the facial area. Here is a simple outline of the technique:

1. **Preparation:** The patient lies comfortably on a massage table, face up, ensuring a relaxed and supported head position. For facial MLD, the therapist will focus on the face and neck regions. The therapist should always commence the session by stimulating the lymph nodes of face and neck that enhances the transport of lymph fluid through the circulatory system.

2. **Gentle Strokes:** The therapist begins with very light, gentle strokes on the face, following specific pathways of the lymphatic system. These strokes are applied with soft pressure to avoid any discomfort or irritation to the delicate facial tissues.

3. **Sequential Movements:** Using specific sequences of movements, the therapist targets key lymphatic drainage areas in the face, such as the cheeks, jawline, and under the chin. Circular and pumping motions are often employed to encourage lymph flow and fluid movement.

4. **Focus on Draining Nodes**: Special attention is given to stimulating the lymph nodes located around the ear and neck regions. These nodes play a crucial role in draining excess fluid from the face. The massage primarily focuses on the face, neck, and clavicle areas, targeting regions with the highest fluid accumulation. Given the presence of swelling and bruising, particularly around incisions located under the earlobe and chin, a gentle approach to massage is essential. Using fingertips, thumbs, and light full-hand strokes, the therapist gently directs the fluid from the face towards the lymph nodes near the earlobes, down the neck, and into the clavicle region.

   Clients who have undergone a facelift procedure often experience noticeable swelling in areas such as the cheeks, under the eyes, and the neck, primarily due to the limited space on the face that makes edema more conspicuous. While the development of fibrotic tissue is usually mild, it tends to be more noticeable around the jaw and neck. In such cases, clients can benefit from self-massage techniques, which can be taught to them to aid in their recovery process.

5. **Avoiding Pressure on Incision Sites:** If the face lift involved incisions, the therapist will take care to avoid applying direct pressure on those areas. The goal is to support fluid drainage without disturbing the healing process.

6. **Post-Treatment Care:** After the session, the therapist may provide instructions for self-care techniques, such as gentle

facial exercises and deep breathing, to further enhance lymphatic drainage between sessions.

Note:

It's essential to note that facial LM requires specialized training and a thorough understanding of facial anatomy. Therefore, it is crucial to seek the expertise of a qualified LM therapist experienced in post-face lift care. They can provide personalized guidance to promote healing, reduce swelling, and support your recovery journey after the surgical procedure.

Tip:

Since the face and neck are relatively small surface areas of the body and easily accessible, self-administered LM can often be performed at home. This provides a convenient and effective way to complement professional LM sessions during your recovery. By asking your LM therapist about techniques and the appropriate frequency of massage that you can do at home, you can actively participate in your healing journey.

Self-administered LM can have significant benefits, especially in terms of facilitating faster resolution of swelling and bruising. By gently and correctly performing the massage techniques at home, you can support the lymphatic system in removing excess fluid and reducing inflammation. This proactive approach can lead to a smoother recovery process and potentially decrease the number of visits you need to make to your therapist.

To ensure that you are performing self-administered LM correctly and safely, your therapist needs to provide you with personalized instructions and guidance. LM specialists can demonstrate the appropriate techniques, taking into consideration the specific surgical procedure you underwent and the areas that require attention. These techniques may include gentle strokes, circular motions, and movements targeted at specific lymph nodes in the face and neck.

Remember that self-administered LM is not meant to replace professional sessions but to complement them. Your therapist will determine the suitable timing and frequency for you to perform the massage at home, ensuring it aligns with your recovery progress. It's crucial to follow their recommendations to avoid any potential complications and to maximize the benefits of self-administered LM.

By actively participating in your recovery with self-administered LM, you can contribute to a more effective healing process and achieve more favorable outcomes after your face and neck procedures. Working in partnership with your therapist and maintaining open communication will empower you to take an active role in your recovery and overall well-being.

LEARN MORE:

Scan or click here to learn more tips for recovery after a face lift.

71

IS LYMPHATIC MASSAGE BENEFICIAL FOR RECOVERY AFTER UPPER EYELID SURGERY (BLEPHAROPLASTY)?

Yes, LM can be beneficial for recovery after upper eyelid surgery (blepharoplasty). Blepharoplasty is a surgical procedure that involves the removal of excess skin, muscle, and fat from the upper eyelids to improve appearance and address issues such as sagging eyelids or puffiness.

After blepharoplasty, some patients may experience swelling and bruising around the eyes, which is a common part of the healing process. MLD can be a helpful therapeutic approach to manage postoperative swelling and enhance the recovery process.

The gentle and precise techniques of MLD can aid in reducing fluid buildup and edema around the eyes. By promoting lymphatic flow, MLD assists the body's natural drainage mechanisms, allowing excess fluid and waste products to be carried away more efficiently. This can help to alleviate swelling and accelerate the healing process.

Note:

It is crucial to consult with your surgeon before incorporating MLD into your postoperative care. They will assess your individual healing progress and provide guidance on the appropriate timing and techniques for MLD after blepharoplasty. Moreover, it's essential to work with a qualified and experienced LM therapist who is familiar with the specific considerations for post-blepharoplasty care.

Overall, MLD can be a valuable addition to your recovery routine after upper eyelid surgery, supporting your body's natural healing processes and promoting a smoother and more comfortable healing journey.

Tip:

One important tip for clients undergoing LM after blepharoplasty is to communicate openly with your LM therapist about any discomfort or sensitivity in the eye area. Since the eye area is delicate and sensitive after the surgery, it's essential to let the therapist know about any specific sensations or concerns you may have during the massage.

LEARN MORE:

Scan or click here to learn more tips for recovery after upper and lower blepharoplasty.

72

WHAT IS THE BASIC TECHNIQUE FOR MANUAL LYMPHATIC DRAINAGE AFTER EYELID SURGERY (BLEPHAROPLASTY)?

After eyelid surgery (blepharoplasty), the basic technique for LM should be gentle and focused on promoting lymphatic flow while avoiding direct pressure on the surgical site. Here is the basic outline of the technique:

1. **Communication:** Before starting MLD, communicate with your client to ensure they are comfortable and have no specific concerns about their eyes or the surgical area. Encourage them to share any sensations or discomfort they may experience during the massage.

2. **Positioning:** To begin the session effectively, the therapist should always start by stimulating the lymph nodes in the face and neck. This stimulation enhances the movement of lymph fluid through the circulatory system.

3. **Gentle Strokes:** The therapist should begin with very light and gentle strokes on the face, following specific pathways of the lymphatic system. They should avoid direct pressure on the eyes and the surgical area. Instead, focus on strokes that move away from the eyes, towards the temples and hairline.

4. **Lymph Node Stimulation:** The therapist should pay special attention to stimulating lymph nodes located around the eyes, such as the pre-auricular and parotid lymph nodes. Gentle circular motions can be used to promote lymphatic drainage in these areas.

5. **Directional Flow:** Use slow and rhythmic movements to facilitate the flow of lymph away from the eyes and towards the lymphatic collectors in the neck and behind the ears.

6. **Avoiding Incision Sites:** Be cautious not to apply pressure on the incision sites or any areas of the face that may still be sensitive from the surgery.

7. **Communication and Feedback:** Throughout the massage, maintain open communication with the client, encouraging them to share any sensations or discomfort. Adjust the technique accordingly to ensure their comfort and safety.

Note:

It's crucial to work with a qualified and experienced LM therapist who is familiar with post-blepharoplasty care. They can tailor the technique to the client's specific needs and ensure that MLD supports their healing process without causing any discomfort or irritation.

Tip:

Typically, after blepharoplasty, incisions are closed with temporary external sutures that need to be removed within three to ten days. It's essential to discuss with both your surgeon and your LM therapist whether LM can be performed while the external sutures are still present, and if so, what specific limitations or precautions should be followed.

Firstly, ensure that your surgeon gives the green light for LM with the external sutures in place. They will assess the healing progress and determine whether it is safe to proceed with the massage. In some cases, the presence of external sutures may require temporarily delaying LM until they are removed to avoid any risk of disrupting the incisions.

If LM is deemed appropriate during the period of external sutures, communicate this information with your LM therapist. They will need to adapt their techniques to work carefully around the sutures and avoid putting any pressure on or around the surgical site. Gentle strokes and focused movements away from the eyes and surgical areas will be emphasized to support lymphatic drainage without interfering with the healing process.

Keep in mind that the area around the eyes is delicate and sensitive, so any massage must be conducted with extreme care and precision. By collaborating closely with both your surgeon and LM therapist, you can ensure that your recovery journey after blepharoplasty is supported in the most effective and safe manner.

Remember, the primary focus during this period is on allowing the incisions to heal properly, so always prioritize the advice and recommendations of your surgical and LM teams. By following their guidance, you can optimize the healing process and achieve the best possible outcomes after your blepharoplasty surgery.

LEARN MORE:

Scan or click <u>here</u> to learn more about the top three oils to use for LM after blepharoplasty.

73

WHAT IS THE BASIC TECHNIQUE FOR MANUAL LYMPHATIC DRAINAGE AFTER NECK LIPOSUCTION?

The basic technique for LM after neck liposuction involves gentle and precise movements to promote lymphatic flow and reduce swelling in the treated area. Here is an outline of the basic technique:

1. **Communication:** Before starting MLD, communicate with the client to understand their specific concerns and ensure they are comfortable with the massage. To initiate the session effectively, the therapist should always start by stimulating the lymph nodes in the face and neck, enhancing the flow of lymphatic fluid through the circulatory system.

2. **Positioning:** Position the client comfortably on a massage table with their head and neck slightly elevated to facilitate lymphatic flow.

3. **Gentle Strokes:** Begin with very light and gentle strokes on the neck, moving in a direction away from the surgical site. Use slow, rhythmic movements to encourage lymphatic drainage.

4. **Neck Lymph Nodes:** Pay special attention to the lymph nodes located in the neck, such as the submandibular and cervical lymph nodes. Use gentle circular motions to stimulate lymphatic flow in these areas.

5. **Directional Flow:** Use strokes that move towards the lymphatic collectors in the neck, behind the ears, and towards the clavicle. This helps direct the lymphatic fluid away from the neck and promotes its drainage.

6. **Avoiding Incision Sites:** Be cautious not to apply pressure on the incision sites or any areas that may still be sensitive from the surgery.

7. **Compression:** Consider using light compression garments or bandages to support the neck and facilitate lymphatic flow. Your surgeon may recommend specific compression techniques or garments for the post-liposuction period.

8. **Hydration:** Encourage the client to stay well-hydrated to support the lymphatic system in effectively removing excess fluid.

9. **Frequency:** The frequency of MLD sessions will depend on the individual's healing progress and the recommendation of their surgeon. Typically, more frequent sessions may be needed in the early postoperative period.

Note:

Always consult with a qualified and experienced LM therapist who is familiar with post-neck liposuction care. They can tailor the technique to your specific needs and ensure that manual lymphatic drainage supports your healing process without causing any discomfort or irritation.

Tip:

For self-administered MLD at home, the neck is an easily accessible area. To facilitate your recovery, ask your LM therapist early on about techniques you can perform at home. They can provide you with guidance and demonstrate the proper strokes and movements to help promote lymphatic flow in the neck area.

Remember to be gentle and use light pressure during self-administered LM. Start with slow and rhythmic strokes, moving away from the front neck and towards the lymphatic collectors in the neck, behind the ears, and towards the clavicle. This will help direct the lymphatic fluid away from the neck and encourage drainage.

LEARN MORE:

Scan or click here to learn more tips for recovery after neck liposuction.

74

DOES LYMPHATIC MASSAGE BENEFIT RECOVERY AFTER SMART LIPOSUCTION?

Yes, LM can benefit recovery after smart liposuction, just like any other liposuction technique. Smart liposuction, also known as laser liposuction or laser-assisted liposuction, uses laser energy to liquefy fat before it is removed through suction. While smart liposuction is designed to be less invasive and cause less trauma compared to traditional liposuction, it still results in the accumulation of fluid and swelling in the treated areas.

LM is a gentle and specialized massage technique that focuses on promoting lymphatic flow and reducing postoperative swelling. After smart liposuction, the body's lymphatic system may become overwhelmed with excess fluid and cellular debris, leading to edema (swelling). LM helps to stimulate the lymphatic system, facilitating the removal of this fluid and cellular waste from the body.

By promoting proper lymphatic drainage, LM can accelerate the healing process, reduce swelling and bruising, and enhance overall recovery after smart liposuction. It can also help to improve the contour and smoothness of the treated areas, leading to better cosmetic results.

Note:

One of the notable benefits of smart liposuction is its ability to reduce the amount of swelling and bruising during the recovery period. This innovative liposuction procedure utilizes laser energy to liquefy fat before removal, causing less trauma to the surrounding tissues compared to traditional liposuction techniques. As a result, patients often experience milder postoperative swelling and bruising, contributing to a more comfortable and smoother recovery process.

However, despite the reduced swelling and bruising, smart liposuction can still impact the lymphatic system similarly, if not more extensively, compared to traditional liposuction. The body's lymphatic system plays a crucial role in removing excess fluid, cellular waste, and toxins from the treated areas. Any disruption to the lymphatic system can hinder the body's natural ability to drain and process these substances, leading to edema (fluid retention) and potentially delaying the healing process.

This is where MLD after smart liposuction becomes especially beneficial. MLD is a specialized massage technique designed to stimulate the lymphatic system, encouraging proper fluid flow and enhancing the body's natural waste removal process. By promoting lymphatic drainage, MLD can effectively reduce postoperative edema, accelerate healing, and enhance overall recovery outcomes.

Tip:

It is crucial to have a clear understanding of the type of liposuction planned for your surgery. Communication with both your surgeon and your LM therapist is essential, as different liposuction methods may require specific LM techniques to optimize the positive effects of LM during your post-surgical recovery.

If you are undergoing smart liposuction, which utilizes laser energy to liquefy fat before removal, it is vital to inform your LM therapist about this technique. Smart liposuction can cause a similar or potentially more extensive impact on the lymphatic system compared to traditional liposuction. As a result, the use of MLD after smart liposuction can be even more beneficial in supporting proper lymphatic flow and reducing postoperative edema.

On the other hand, traditional liposuction techniques may involve more direct mechanical disruption of fat cells, resulting in different healing processes and lymphatic challenges. In such cases, your LM therapist may need to adjust their techniques accordingly to effectively address the specific needs of traditional liposuction recovery.

By discussing the planned liposuction technique with your LM therapist, they can tailor their approach to your unique situation, ensuring that MLD is performed in a way that optimizes its benefits for your post-surgical recovery. This proactive communication between your surgeon and LM therapist will help to create a cohesive and effective postoperative care plan, leading to a smoother and more successful recovery process.

Remember, the goal of incorporating MLD after liposuction is to promote lymphatic drainage, reduce swelling, and enhance overall healing. With a well-informed and collaborative approach, you can maximize the positive impact of LM on your recovery journey and achieve the best possible outcomes from your liposuction procedure.

LEARN MORE:

Scan or click here to learn more about the difference between regular and SMART liposuction.

75

Is lymphatic massage different for recovery after CoolSculpting compared to regular liposuction?

Yes, LM techniques and approach for recovery after CoolSculpting can be different compared to traditional liposuction. While both procedures aim to reduce unwanted fat, they work in different ways and have distinct effects on the body's lymphatic system.

Note:

CoolSculpting is a non-invasive fat reduction procedure that uses controlled cooling to target and freeze fat cells, causing them to undergo apoptosis (cell death). The body then naturally eliminates these dead fat cells over time through the lymphatic system. Unlike traditional liposuction, CoolSculpting does not involve surgical incisions or direct mechanical disruption of fat cells.

Due to the non-invasive nature of CoolSculpting, the recovery period is generally less intensive compared to traditional liposuction.

However, the process of eliminating the frozen fat cells through the lymphatic system can still lead to some post-treatment swelling and discomfort.

MLD after CoolSculpting focuses on facilitating the lymphatic system's natural drainage process to help remove the processed fat cells efficiently. The MLD techniques used may involve gentle strokes and movements that encourage lymphatic flow in the treated areas. The goal is to minimize swelling and promote the body's ability to flush out the destroyed fat cells, leading to enhanced and more comfortable recovery.

On the other hand, after traditional liposuction, MLD aims to address the impact of the surgical procedure on the lymphatic system. The technique may involve more specific and targeted strokes to assist with fluid drainage, reduce postoperative edema, and optimize overall healing.

Tip:

Indeed, the recovery after CoolSculpting may require additional effort in restoring lymphatic outflow from the treated areas. While CoolSculpting is a non-invasive procedure, it still impacts the lymphatic system as the body works to eliminate the processed fat cells. As a result, some individuals may experience increased swelling or edema in the treated areas, which can affect the lymphatic flow.

To address this, MLD sessions may need to be more frequent and longer in duration. The goal of MLD after CoolSculpting is to facilitate the body's natural lymphatic drainage process, helping to reduce swelling and promote the efficient removal of the treated fat cells.

LEARN MORE:

Scan or click here to learn more about the difference between Coolscupting and regular liposuction.

76

WHAT IS FIBROSIS AFTER LIPOSUCTION?

Fibrosis after liposuction refers to the formation of scar tissue or fibrous tissue in the treated area as part of the body's healing response. Liposuction is a surgical procedure that involves the removal of excess fat from specific body areas. While it is generally considered safe and effective, liposuction can cause trauma to the surrounding tissues, including blood vessels, nerves, and lymphatic vessels.

As a natural part of the healing process, the body attempts to repair the damaged tissues by laying down collagen fibers, which form scar tissue. In some cases, excessive scar tissue can develop in the treated area, leading to fibrosis. Fibrosis can cause the tissues to become thickened, hardened, and less flexible, leading to discomfort and an altered appearance in the treated area.

Fibrosis can manifest as areas of firmness, lumpiness, or unevenness under the skin after liposuction. While mild fibrosis is relatively common and may resolve on its own with time, more significant fibrosis can be problematic and may require medical attention.

Manual lymphatic drainage (MLD) is one of the techniques used to address fibrosis after liposuction. MLD is a specialized massage technique that focuses on stimulating the lymphatic system to reduce swelling, promote fluid drainage, and improve the healing process. By encouraging lymphatic flow, MLD can help to alleviate fibrosis and improve the overall appearance and comfort of the treated area.

Note:

Fibrosis post-liposuction can manifest in two forms: diffuse or local. Diffuse fibrosis occurs after overly aggressive liposuction, affecting large areas (such as the flanks or stomach), leading to a firm, hard, and inflexible "leathery-like" surface. In contrast, local fibrosis appears as a small, tender lump palpable over the liposuction area, representing a small, concentrated zone of increased fibrosis within the healing tissue. Local fibrosis is often detectable once initial swelling subsides, typically within one to three weeks after surgery.

One of the major benefits of LM is the prevention of fibrosis areas. Eliminating excessive fluid and reducing inflammation in the surgical area with LM techniques optimizes healing properties of the surgical sites which prevents the development of excessive scar tissue that can lead to fibrosis.

Tip:

Preventing fibrosis after liposuction is crucial for achieving optimal postoperative results. One of the most effective ways to do this is by incorporating early and regular MLD.

Early in your treatment sessions, consult with your LM therapist about recognizing signs of fibrotic areas. They can also instruct you on specific self-massage techniques that you can practice at home to prevent or mitigate fibrous areas.

Early initiation of MLD after liposuction can help kickstart the body's natural healing processes, including the lymphatic system. MLD techniques focus on gently stimulating the lymphatic vessels to improve fluid circulation, reduce swelling, and promote the elimination of cellular debris and excess fluids from the treated area. By encouraging the proper flow of lymph, MLD can help prevent the buildup of fibrous tissue and reduce the risk of developing fibrosis.

Regular MLD sessions are equally important as they maintain the ongoing benefits of improved lymphatic flow. Consistent MLD helps prevent stagnation of fluid, which could contribute to fibrosis over time. Frequent sessions in the early postoperative period can be particularly helpful in reducing swelling and promoting proper tissue healing.

Ask your LM therapist to identify any areas of fibrosis that may be developing and address them promptly. Early detection allows for more targeted interventions and a higher likelihood of successful fibrosis management.

LEARN MORE:

Scan or click here to learn more about fibrosis formation after liposuction.

77

HOW DO I KNOW IF I HAVE FIBROSIS?

Fibrosis after liposuction can indeed present as firm and tender lumps under the skin, which can be uncomfortable and sometimes painful. These lumps may vary in size and can be located at different depths within the treated area. Fibrosis typically begins to develop in the early postoperative period, usually around one to three weeks after liposuction surgery.

Without proper treatment, fibrosis may persist for an extended period and may not completely resolve on its own. During the resolution of fibrosis, individuals may continue to experience pain and discomfort in the affected area, which can be bothersome and impact daily activities.

Early intervention with manual lymphatic drainage (MLD) can significantly aid in preventing or minimizing the development of fibrosis. MLD focuses on promoting lymphatic flow and reducing swelling, which can help prevent fluid stagnation and the accumulation of fibrous tissue. Regular MLD sessions in the early postoperative period can also help identify and address fibrosis promptly, leading to a more comfortable and successful recovery.

If fibrosis does occur, therapeutic MLD techniques can still be beneficial in managing the condition and improving overall tissue health. While fibrosis may take time to subside completely, ongoing MLD treatment can aid in reducing discomfort and improving the appearance and feel of the treated area.

It is essential to work closely with a qualified and experienced MLD therapist who can tailor the treatment to your specific needs and provide the best possible care during your liposuction recovery. By addressing fibrosis proactively and seeking early treatment, you can enhance the healing process and optimize your postoperative outcomes.

Note:

The body's natural healing processes, including lymphatic drainage and tissue remodeling, play a crucial role in resolving fibrosis. Smaller areas of fibrosis are more manageable for the body to address, and with the help of manual lymphatic drainage (MLD) and other therapeutic interventions, they can heal more efficiently.

However, larger fibrotic areas may require more time for the body to break down and reabsorb the excess collagen and scar tissue. These areas can be more resistant to treatment, and it may take several months for them to fully subside.

Early intervention with MLD and other appropriate treatments can play a significant role in managing fibrosis regardless of its size. The goal is to promote proper lymphatic flow, reduce swelling, and stimulate tissue healing, ultimately supporting the resolution of fibrotic areas.

Tip:

The earlier fibrosis is diagnosed, and the earlier fibrosis treatment can be started the faster it disappears. In order to diagnose potential fibrosis, constantly palpate your liposuction areas and try to feel any lumps or bumps. If you notice anything suspicious, show the area to your LM therapist so that if fibrosis is confirmed, you can start treatment as soon as possible.

 **LEARN MORE:**

Scan or click here to discover more ways to diagnose fibrosis.

78

WHAT HAPPENS IF FIBROSIS DOSE NOT RESOLVE?

If left untreated, fibrosis areas can persist for a long time and may eventually become palpable as a scar under the skin. While the pain associated with fibrosis usually resolves over time, the palpable lumps may decrease in size but still remain. If there is no change in the size of the fibrosis area after six months to a year, it is unlikely to naturally resolve, and a permanent thick scar may have formed. In such cases, it is essential to discuss the condition with your surgeon to explore potential treatment options.

There are several ways to address permanent fibrosis. Some of the available treatments include steroid injections, excision, liposuction, fat grafting, and others. Each option should be carefully considered and discussed with your surgeon to determine the most suitable approach for your specific case.

Note:

It is important to note that treating fibrosis requires time, effort, and patience. For faster and more effective results, incorporating specialized techniques during MLD sessions and additional measures at home can be beneficial. Techniques such as using heating pads, focused vibration massage, and stretching of surrounding tissues can complement MLD and aid in the resolution of fibrosis.

Tip:

It is essential to communicate any potential fibrosis areas you've noticed to your surgeon. Even if the fibrosis is being treated by an MLD therapist, your surgeon should be informed about these areas. This communication is crucial to ensure that your surgeon is aware of the progress of fibrosis and can closely monitor its resolution.

While MLD can be effective in addressing fibrosis, some cases may require additional intervention. If fibrosis persists despite MLD treatment, your surgeon may need to consider other options, such as steroid injections, excision, liposuction, or fat grafting, to achieve the best possible outcome.

By keeping your surgeon informed, you create a collaborative approach to your postoperative care. Your surgeon can work in conjunction with your MLD therapist to ensure the most comprehensive and effective treatment plan for addressing fibrosis. Regular follow-up appointments with your surgeon will allow them to assess the progress of fibrosis and determine if any further action is needed.

Remember that every individual's response to surgery and recovery is unique, and fibrosis can vary in its presentation and resolution. By maintaining open communication with both your surgeon and MLD therapist, you can ensure that any fibrosis concerns are addressed promptly and effectively, leading to a smoother and more successful recovery journey.

LEARN MORE:

Scan or click <u>here</u> to learn about additional options to treat fibrosis after liposuction.

79

WHAT ARE THE MASSAGE TECHNIQUES TO TREAT FIBROSIS AREAS?

Massage techniques to treat fibrosis areas involve targeted and specific manual manipulation of the affected tissues to break down scar tissue and promote lymphatic flow. Here are some common massage techniques used to address fibrosis:

1. **MLD:** This is a gentle, rhythmic massage technique designed to stimulate the lymphatic system and encourage the removal of excess fluid and waste products. MLD helps to reduce swelling and inflammation in the fibrosis area and aids in the reabsorption of scar tissue.

2. **Cross-Friction Massage:** This technique involves applying deep pressure and friction perpendicular to the direction of the fibrotic tissue fibers. Cross-friction massage helps break down adhesions and scar tissue, promoting tissue flexibility and improved range of motion.

3. **Trigger Point Therapy:** This involves applying pressure to specific trigger points, or knots, in the muscles to release tension and improve blood flow. This technique can help alleviate pain and discomfort associated with fibrosis.

4. **Deep Tissue Massage:** This targets the deeper layers of muscles and connective tissue to break down adhesions and scar tissue. This technique can help improve circulation and reduce fibrosis.

5. **Instrument-Assisted Massage:** Some therapists may use specialized tools or instruments to apply pressure and break down fibrosis more effectively.

6. **Stretching and Range of Motion Exercises:** Gentle stretching and range of motion exercises can help improve tissue flexibility and prevent further adhesions.

7. **Cupping Therapy:** This is effective in breaking down fibrotic tissue, especially after the initial healing phase. Its benefits include elevating tissues, improving blood circulation, and aiding in toxin release. However, it's essential to use this therapy cautiously during early recovery stages to prevent potential complications. This technique, notable for its suction, helps loosen fibrotic areas, enhances healing through better blood flow, and stimulates lymphatic drainage, thereby removing bodily toxins.

Note:

Heat therapy can be beneficial for fibrosis resolution, but it should be used with caution and only after consulting with your surgeon or healthcare professional. After surgery, the skin's sensitivity may be altered, and the application of warm heating pads, which are generally safe for healthy skin, may cause discomfort or even burns in the treated areas. Therefore, it is essential to discuss the use of heating pads over liposuction areas with your doctor before implementing this technique.

If your surgeon approves the use of heating pads, follow their guidelines for safe and effective application. Make sure to choose a heating pad that allows you to control the temperature and avoid using it at a level that might cause discomfort or harm. Additionally, do not apply heating pads directly on areas with reduced sensitivity or numbness after surgery, as you may not feel any potential damage or irritation.

It's crucial to be mindful of any changes in skin sensation and report any discomfort or adverse reactions to your healthcare provider immediately. Combining heat therapy with other massage techniques can be a comprehensive approach to treating fibrosis and promoting healing after liposuction surgery. Always prioritize your safety and follow the guidance of your medical team throughout the recovery process.

Tip:

Secondary heat conduction can be a helpful technique to apply heat to fibrosis areas with lower risks of thermal injury. To perform this technique, start by holding a warm pad in your hands for a few minutes to warm up your palms. Be cautious not to overheat the pad or your hands, ensuring they feel comfortable to the touch. Once your hands are warm, place them gently over the fibrosis area and allow the heat to penetrate for a few minutes.

This method allows you to control the heat intensity and avoid direct contact with the heating pad on sensitive or numb areas. The gentle warmth from your hands can be soothing and help improve blood flow, which aids in softening and breaking down fibrosis.

For an added effect, you can apply some gentle massage to the area while maintaining the warmth of your hands. Gentle massage can help stimulate circulation and promote fluid movement, further aiding in the resolution of fibrosis.

LEARN MORE:

Scan or click here for insights on identifying improvements in fibrosis with treatment.

80

WILL FIBROSIS POST-LIPOSUCTION RESOLVE ON ITS OWN?

Fibrosis after liposuction may improve and soften over time, but in some cases, it may not completely go away. The resolution of fibrosis depends on various factors, such as the individual's healing response, the extent of fibrosis, and the effectiveness of the treatment provided.

With proper care and management, fibrosis can gradually diminish, especially with early intervention, consistent LM and other therapeutic techniques. LM helps to promote fluid movement and tissue healing, which can aid in breaking down fibrotic tissue and reducing its impact on the surrounding area.

However, larger or more established fibrotic areas may be more challenging to resolve completely. In such cases, additional treatments, like specialized massage techniques, focused ultrasound, or surgical interventions, may be considered to address persistent fibrosis.

Note:

It is essential to work closely with your surgeon and LM therapist to monitor the progress of fibrosis and determine the best course of action for your individual case. Early detection and proactive management can improve the chances of fibrosis resolution and promote a smoother recovery after liposuction.

Tip:

Communication with your surgeon about any concerns regarding fibrosis is crucial during follow-up visits. If you notice areas of fibrosis or experience any symptoms that may indicate its presence, be sure to point them out to your surgeon. Describe the symptoms and the location of the fibrotic areas to the best of your ability.

Your surgeon is the best person to diagnose and assess the condition. They can determine if the firmness or tenderness you are experiencing is indeed fibrosis and provide appropriate guidance on how to manage it. Depending on the severity and extent of fibrosis, your surgeon may recommend specific treatments or techniques to help soften and resolve the fibrotic areas.

Early detection and timely intervention can play a significant role in addressing fibrosis effectively. By working closely with your surgeon and following their advice, you can take proactive steps towards promoting a smoother recovery and achieving the best possible outcomes after liposuction or any other surgical procedure.

 **LEARN MORE:**

Scan or click here to learn about the stages of fibrosis development and treatment options for each stage.

81

WHAT IS THE BEST OIL FOR LYMPHATIC MASSAGE AND FIBROSIS?

The choice of oil for LM and fibrosis can vary based on personal preference, individual needs, and any potential allergies or sensitivities. There are no one-size-fits-all answers as different oils offer unique benefits. Here are some commonly used oils for LM and fibrosis:

1. **Coconut Oil:** This is known for its moisturizing properties and is often used in LM. It is easily absorbed by the skin and can help improve lymphatic flow.

2. **Jojoba Oil:** This closely resembles the skin's natural sebum, making it an excellent choice for massage. It is non-comedogenic and suitable for all skin types.

3. **Sweet Almond Oil:** This is rich in vitamins and has anti-inflammatory properties, making it beneficial for LM and reducing inflammation associated with fibrosis.

4. **Grapeseed Oil:** This is a light and non-greasy oil that is easily absorbed by the skin. It is suitable for sensitive skin and can help improve lymphatic circulation.

5. **Arnica Oil:** This is derived from the arnica flower and is known for its anti-inflammatory properties. It can be beneficial for reducing swelling and bruising associated with fibrosis.

6. **Calendula Oil:** This is derived from marigold flowers and is often used for its anti-inflammatory and healing properties. It can be helpful for promoting tissue repair in fibrosis areas.

Note:

While these oils are popular choices, it is essential to consider individual factors such as skin type, allergies, and medical history before selecting an LM oil. As the market continues to expand, it's a good idea to keep an eye out for new and specialized oils specifically formulated for LM and fibrosis management. Always consult with a qualified LM therapist or healthcare professional to determine the most suitable LM oil for your unique needs.

Tip:

Creating your own LM oil using coconut oil and essential oils of lavender, arnica, and grapefruit is simple and effective. Here's the basic recipe to get you started:

Ingredients:

- 1/2 cup of liquid coconut oil
- 5 drops of lavender essential oil
- 5 drops of arnica essential oil
- 5 drops of grapefruit essential oil

Remember to perform a patch test before using this LM oil on a larger area to ensure you don't have any allergic reactions or skin sensitivities to the essential oils. If you experience any irritation, discontinue use and consult with a healthcare professional.

LEAN MORE:

Scan or click <u>here</u> to find more recipes for LM oils.

82

WHAT IS THE BASIC TECHNIQUE FOR SELF-MASSAGE OF A SMALL FIBROSIS AREA?

Performing self-massage on small fibrosis areas can be beneficial in promoting fluid movement and reducing discomfort. Here's the basic technique you can try:

1. **Preparation:** Wash your hands thoroughly to ensure they are clean before touching the affected area. You may also apply a small amount of the DIY LM oil (coconut oil with essential oils) we discussed earlier to the fibrosis area for added lubrication.

2. **Gentle Pressure:** Use your fingertips to apply gentle pressure on the fibrosis area. Start with very light pressure and gradually increase it as you become more comfortable.

3. **Circular Motion:** Using small circular motions, gently massage the fibrosis area. Imagine drawing small circles with your fingers on the skin. Avoid pressing too hard to prevent any additional discomfort.

4. **Directional Strokes:** After performing circular motions for a few minutes, switch to gentle directional strokes. Start from the edges of the fibrosis and stroke towards the nearest lymph nodes. For example, if the fibrosis is on your arm, stroke towards the underarm lymph nodes.

5. **Stretching:** To further encourage fluid movement, perform gentle stretching movements in the surrounding areas. For instance, if the fibrosis is on your thigh, gently stretch and bend your knee.

6. **Repeat:** Continue the self-massage for about five to ten minutes, focusing on the fibrosis area and its surrounding tissues.

7. **Rest:** After the self-massage, take a few moments to rest and relax. You can also elevate the affected limb to further aid fluid drainage.

8. **Consistency:** Perform this self-massage technique regularly, ideally once or twice a day, to help reduce the fibrosis and promote better lymphatic flow.

Note:

In addition to manual massage, using a special fibrosis massager can provide further assistance in resolving this problematic area. A round hand-held roller massager is an excellent option as it is easy to use and comfortable to operate. This type of massager is designed to target specific areas of fibrosis with gentle yet effective pressure, helping to break down the fibrous tissues and promote better lymphatic flow.

When using the fibrosis massager, start with light pressure and gradually increase it as you become more accustomed to the sensation. Gently roll the massager over the affected area in small circular motions or along the direction of lymphatic drainage, following the techniques discussed earlier. The massager's rolling action helps to stimulate the lymphatic system, encouraging fluid movement and facilitating the resolution of fibrosis.

Using a fibrosis massager can be a convenient and beneficial addition to your self-care routine. Regularly incorporating this tool into your post-surgery recovery plan, along with manual massage and other recommended techniques, can contribute to a faster and more effective resolution of fibrosis.

Before using a fibrosis massager or any other medical device, be sure to consult with your healthcare professional or LM therapist. They can provide specific guidance on how to use the massager correctly and tailor it to your individual needs and condition.

Tip:

For more information about fibrosis massagers and their potential benefits, you can explore the provided link to find the best options available. Remember that consistent and safe application of these tools, in conjunction with professional advice, can greatly support your recovery journey and improve your overall well-being.

LEARN MORE:

Scan or click here to learn more about the benefits of using a fibrosis massager.

83

WHAT IS THE BASIC TECHNIQUE FOR SELF-MASSAGE OF A LARGE FIBROSIS AREA?

Self-massage of a large fibrosis area requires gentle yet consistent pressure to promote the breakdown of fibrous tissues and facilitate better lymphatic drainage. Here's the basic technique you can use:

1. **Warm-up:** Before starting the massage, apply a warm compress or use a heating pad on the fibrosis area for a few minutes. This helps to increase blood flow and makes the tissues more pliable, making the massage more effective.

2. **Lubricate:** Apply a small amount of LM oil or any suitable massage oil to the skin over the fibrosis area. This helps reduce friction during the massage and makes the movements smoother.

3. **Circular Strokes:** Using the pads of your fingers, gently apply pressure in small circular motions over the fibrosis area. Start with light pressure and gradually increase it if it

feels comfortable. Be mindful not to apply excessive force, as it may cause discomfort or aggravate the condition.

4. **Long Strokes:** After using circular strokes, switch to longer, sweeping strokes along the direction of lymphatic drainage. This typically involves moving the fingers in an upward direction towards the nearest lymph nodes. The goal is to encourage fluid movement and help drain excess fluid from the fibrosis area.

5. **Repeat:** Continue massaging the fibrosis area for five to ten minutes, taking short breaks as needed. Consistency is key, so try to incorporate self-massage into your daily routine, especially if you have a large fibrosis area.

6. **Cooling Down:** After the massage, apply a cool compress or use a cooling pad on the area for a few minutes. This helps to reduce any potential inflammation caused by the massage.

Note:

Remember to be patient with the self-massage process, as it may take time to see significant improvements in large fibrosis areas. If you experience any pain or discomfort during the self-massage, stop immediately and consult with your healthcare professional or LM therapist for further guidance.

Always seek professional advice before attempting self-massage on a large fibrosis area to ensure that the technique is safe and appropriate for your specific condition and needs.

Post liposuction body massagers are highly effective in treating large fibrosis areas on the abdomen, flanks, and back. These specialized devices offer comprehensive massage coverage over significant surface areas, making the treatment process effortless and efficient.

These massagers are specifically designed to address fibrosis, helping to break down stubborn fibrous tissues that can develop after liposuction procedures. By using targeted vibrations and pressure, the massager stimulates circulation, encourages lymphatic drainage, and promotes tissue healing.

The convenience of using a post liposuction body massager lies in its ease of application. With minimal effort, you can massage large areas, ensuring that the affected tissues receive the necessary attention for effective resolution of fibrosis. The gentle yet powerful vibrations of the massager work deep into the tissues, helping to relieve discomfort and improve the overall appearance of the treated areas.

Incorporating the use of a post liposuction body massager into your recovery routine can significantly enhance the results of your liposuction procedure and expedite the healing process. As with any treatment, it's essential to consult with your healthcare professional or LM therapist before using such a device to ensure it is safe and appropriate for your specific condition and needs.

Tip:

Consult your lymphatic massage therapist about at-home massagers ideal for lymphatic drainage and fibrosis management.

LEARN MORE:

Scan or click here to learn more about benefits of an LM roller.

84

WHAT MASSAGERS CAN BE USED
FOR FIBROSIS AREAS?

Several types of massagers can be used to treat fibrosis areas effectively. Here are some common massagers that can help in resolving fibrosis:

1. **Handheld Roller Massagers:** These are versatile and easy to use. They usually have small, rounded knobs or rollers that can be gently applied to the fibrosis area, providing targeted pressure and massage.

2. **Percussion Massagers:** These use rapid, repetitive movements to penetrate deep into the tissues, helping to break down fibrous tissues and promote circulation.

3. **Vibrating Massagers:** These emit gentle vibrations that can be applied to the fibrosis area to stimulate blood flow, reduce inflammation, and promote healing.

4. **Pneumatic Compression Devices:** These devices use air pressure to massage and compress the affected area, facilitating lymphatic drainage and fluid removal.

5. **Ultrasound Massagers:** These use high-frequency sound waves to penetrate the tissues, providing deep therapeutic effects and aiding in the breakdown of fibrosis.

6. **Heat Therapy Devices:** Applying heat to the fibrosis area using heating pads or infrared devices can help relax the tissues and improve circulation, supporting fibrosis resolution.

7. **Foam Rollers:** These can be used to apply pressure and massage large muscle groups, including fibrosis areas in the legs and buttocks.

Note:

When using massagers for fibrosis areas, it's crucial to start with gentle pressure and gradually increase as tolerated. Always consult with your healthcare professional or LM therapist before using any massager to ensure it is safe and suitable for your specific condition and needs. Additionally, it is essential to follow any specific instructions or guidelines provided by your healthcare professional or therapist for the best results and safety during your recovery process.

Tip:

Your LM therapist is likely to have a few massage tools that they can recommend for you to use at home. Don't hesitate to ask them about their recommendations and how to use these tools effectively. It's essential to be well-informed and comfortable with any new massage tool you plan to use, so consider discussing it with your LM therapist beforehand. They can provide valuable insights into whether the massager is suitable for your specific needs and recovery process.

LEARN MORE:

Scan or click <u>here</u> to learn about various massagers to treat fibrosis.

85

CAN A VIBRATING MASSAGER BE USED FOR LYMPHATIC MASSAGE?

Yes, vibrating massagers can be used for LM, and they can be quite effective in promoting lymphatic flow and reducing edema. Vibrating massagers work by creating rapid vibrations that penetrate into the soft tissues, stimulating blood circulation and lymphatic flow.

When using a vibrating massager for LM, it's essential to use the right technique and pressure to avoid any adverse effects. Here are some tips for using a vibrating massager for LM:

1. Use a gentle setting: Set the vibrating massager to a gentle or low intensity setting, especially when targeting areas with lymphatic congestion or fibrosis. Avoid using high intensity or aggressive settings that may cause discomfort or irritation.

2. Direction of massage: Always massage towards the lymph nodes and major lymphatic drainage areas. For example, if you are massaging the legs, massage towards the inguinal lymph nodes located in the groin area.

3. Avoid bony areas: Be cautious not to apply the vibrating massager over bony areas, as this can cause discomfort and may not be effective in stimulating lymphatic flow.

4. Combine with manual techniques: Vibrating massagers can complement manual lymphatic drainage techniques performed by a trained therapist. Using both methods can provide more comprehensive and effective lymphatic support.

5. Use with proper guidance: If you are using a vibrating massager at home, consult with your LM therapist or healthcare professional to ensure you are using the device correctly and safely, especially if you have specific postoperative concerns or conditions.

Note:

Various massage tools are recommended at different stages of post-surgical recovery. In the initial phases, when tissues are tender, manual massage is typically preferred. As healing progresses, hand-held non-vibrating massagers can be introduced to enhance lymphatic flow. By three to six weeks post-surgery, vibrating massagers may be introduced. Electric vibrating massagers can be particularly beneficial in aiding recovery. They offer an intense localized massage that can be especially effective for areas with fibrosis. However, many such massagers are designed for athletic use and may deliver intense vibrations. It's essential to use them judiciously, ensuring they are not introduced too early in the recovery process and are used in a controlled manner to avoid discomfort.

Tip:

Although vibrating massagers are very effective, it's important to exercise caution when choosing the right type for your recovery after surgery. For example, some models, like the gun-type massager, can be too intense and may cause discomfort or tissue damage, even when used on minimal settings, especially during the early stages of the recovery period. It's best to opt for hand-held massagers during the initial and mid-recovery phases, as they allow for better control and are generally gentler on the tissues.

Hand-held massagers are a suitable option for postoperative self-massage, as they provide a more controlled and targeted approach. These types of massagers often have adjustable settings, allowing you to tailor the intensity to your comfort level. They can help reduce muscle tension, promote blood circulation, and gently stimulate lymphatic flow to aid in the resolution of fibrosis and swelling.

As your recovery progresses and your body heals, you can consider incorporating vibration massagers into your self-massage routine. By this time, the tissues may be more resilient, making the vibration therapy better tolerated. Vibration massagers can offer deeper penetration into the muscles, aiding in the release of tension and promoting overall relaxation.

Regardless of the type of vibrating massager you choose, always consult with your healthcare professional or LM therapist before using one. They can provide guidance on the appropriate timing, frequency, and technique to ensure that you use the massager safely and effectively for your specific recovery needs.

It's worth noting that while vibrating massagers can be a beneficial addition to your recovery routine, they should not replace manual lymphatic drainage techniques performed by a trained therapist. Relying on the expertise and specialized techniques of an LM therapist are essential for optimal results and a safe recovery after surgery. Combining both self-massage with vibrating massagers and professional LM can enhance your overall recovery experience and improve the outcomes of your postoperative journey.

243

LEARN MORE:

Scan or click here to learn more about benefits of vibrating massagers.

86

WHAT ELSE CAN HELP WITH RESOLUTION OF FIBROSIS AREAS BESIDES MASSAGE?

In addition to massage, there are several other techniques and measures that can help with the resolution of fibrosis areas:

1. **Heat Therapy:** Applying heat to the fibrosis area can help to increase blood circulation and promote lymphatic drainage. You can use warm compresses or heating pads, but always make sure to check with your surgeon or healthcare professional before using heat therapy to ensure it's safe for your specific situation.

2. **Compression Garments:** Wearing compression garments can aid in reducing swelling and promoting fluid drainage from the fibrosis area. These garments provide gentle pressure on the tissues, helping to prevent the accumulation of excess fluid and supporting the healing process.

3. **Exercises:** Gentle exercises and movement can also be beneficial for resolving fibrosis. Physical activity helps to

stimulate blood flow and lymphatic drainage, preventing stiffness and promoting tissue healing.

4. **Nutrition and Hydration:** A well-balanced diet and adequate hydration are essential for promoting overall healing and reducing inflammation. Make sure to consume a variety of nutrients and drink plenty of water to support your body's recovery.

5. **Topical Creams or Gels:** These may be recommended by your healthcare professional to reduce inflammation and improve tissue healing. Always consult with your surgeon or healthcare provider before using any topical products on the fibrosis area.

6. **Elevation:** Raising the affected area can help with fluid drainage and reduce swelling. For example, if you have fibrosis in your lower extremities, elevating your legs while resting can be beneficial.

7. **Avoiding Certain Activities:** Depending on the location and severity of the fibrosis, your healthcare professional may recommend avoiding certain activities that could exacerbate the condition. This might include avoiding strenuous exercise or activities that put excessive pressure on the affected area.

8. **Additional Modalities:** In some cases, healthcare professionals may recommend other treatment modalities, such as ultrasound therapy or low-level laser therapy, to aid in fibrosis resolution. These therapies should always be conducted under the guidance of a trained professional.

Note:

Incorporating a wide range of fibrosis treatment modalities can indeed lead to faster resolution and improved tissue recovery. Working closely with your LM therapist to explore the various options mentioned earlier can be highly beneficial. Your therapist can provide valuable insights into which techniques may work best for your unique situation and tailor the approach to address your specific needs.

During your discussions with your LM therapist, don't hesitate to ask for precise instructions and directions for each modality. Understanding the correct techniques and methods is crucial to ensure that you apply them effectively at home. Your therapist can demonstrate these techniques, guide you through the process, and address any questions or concerns you may have.

TIP:

Consistency and persistence are key when implementing these treatment modalities. Regularly practicing the techniques at home, as advised by your LM therapist, can significantly contribute to the success of your fibrosis resolution journey. Be patient with the process, as fibrosis recovery may take time, especially for larger or more extensive areas. The combination of professional LM sessions and diligent self-care at home can lead to more rapid and comprehensive results.

LEARN MORE:

Scan or click here to learn about safe application of heating pads after surgery.

87

WHAT SUPPLEMENTS HELP TO DECREASE FIBROSIS?

There are several supplements that are believed to help decrease fibrosis or improve tissue healing after surgery. It is important to note that while some people may find these supplements beneficial, there is limited scientific evidence to support their effectiveness in treating fibrosis. Always consult with your healthcare provider before starting any supplements, especially if you are recovering from surgery. Some supplements that are commonly suggested to potentially aid in reducing fibrosis include:

1. **Bromelain:** An enzyme found in pineapples, bromelain is believed to have anti-inflammatory properties and may help reduce swelling and inflammation.

2. **Arnica Montana:** This herbal supplement is often used to reduce bruising and swelling after surgery and may also have anti-inflammatory effects.

3. **Vitamin C:** An essential nutrient for collagen production, vitamin C may support tissue repair and reduce scar formation.

4. **Vitamin E:** Known for its antioxidant properties, vitamin E may help protect tissues from oxidative stress and support wound healing.

5. **Omega-3 Fatty Acids:** Found in fish oil and flaxseed oil, omega-3 fatty acids have anti-inflammatory properties that may aid in reducing inflammation and fibrosis.

6. **Turmeric/Curcumin:** Curcumin, the active compound in turmeric, is believed to have anti-inflammatory and antioxidant effects, potentially supporting tissue healing.

7. **Gotu Kola:** This traditional herbal supplement is thought to promote collagen production and may assist in wound healing.

8. **N-acetylcysteine (NAC):** This is a precursor to glutathione, a potent antioxidant, and may help reduce oxidative stress and inflammation.

9. **Silica:** This is a mineral that plays a role in collagen formation and may support tissue repair and flexibility.

Note:

Serrapeptase, also known as Serratiopeptidase, is a proteolytic enzyme derived from the bacteria Serratia marcescens. It is believed to have anti-inflammatory and fibrinolytic properties, meaning it may help reduce inflammation and break down excessive fibrin, a protein involved in scar tissue formation. As a result, some people believe that Serrapeptase may be beneficial in treating fibrosis after cosmetic surgery. However, it is important to note that scientific evidence supporting these claims is limited, and more research is needed to establish its effectiveness definitively.

Tip:

It is essential to remember that individual responses to supplements can vary, and their effectiveness may depend on factors like dosage, overall health, and surgical procedure. Always discuss any supplements you are considering with your healthcare provider to ensure they are safe and appropriate for your specific situation.

LEARN MORE:

Scan or click here to learn more about the benefits of Serrapeptase for treatment of fibrosis.

88

WHAT CREAMS OR OILS CAN HELP REDUCE FIBROSIS?

There are several creams and oils that are often recommended to help reduce fibrosis or scar tissue after cosmetic surgery. These products are believed to have anti-inflammatory and moisturizing properties, which may support the healing process and help soften scar tissue. However, it is important to note that while some individuals may find these products beneficial, scientific evidence supporting their effectiveness is limited. Always consult with your healthcare provider or surgeon before using any creams or oils after surgery to ensure they are safe and appropriate for your specific situation. Some common creams and oils that are suggested for reducing fibrosis include:

1. **Silicone Gel:** This is a popular choice for scar management, as it forms a protective barrier over the scar and helps to retain moisture, which may improve the appearance and texture of the scar.

2. **Vitamin E Oil:** This is believed to have antioxidant properties, which may help with tissue healing and scar

reduction. Applying vitamin E oil to the scarred area may help improve its appearance.

3. **Aloe Vera Gel:** This has anti-inflammatory properties and is known for its soothing effect on the skin. Applying aloe vera gel to the scarred area may help reduce inflammation and promote healing.

4. **Cocoa Butter:** This is a rich moisturizer that may help soften scar tissue and improve skin elasticity.

5. **Arnica Cream:** This is derived from the arnica plant and is believed to have anti-inflammatory properties. It is sometimes used to help reduce bruising and swelling after surgery.

6. **Calendula Cream:** This is made from the petals of the marigold flower and is known for its skin-soothing properties. It may be helpful in reducing inflammation and promoting wound healing.

7. **Coconut Oil:** This is a natural moisturizer that can be applied to the skin to help keep it hydrated and supple.

Note:

Remember that individual responses to these creams and oils can vary, and not all products may be suitable for everyone. Always conduct a patch test before applying any new product to a larger area of the skin and discontinue use if you experience any irritation or adverse reactions. Additionally, do not apply any creams or oils to open wounds or incisions until they are fully healed and their use has been approved by your healthcare provider.

Tip:

There are several commercially available topical medications, such as creams and oils, specifically designed to treat fibrosis. These products often contain ingredients that are believed to have anti-inflammatory and collagen-reducing properties, which can help to break down and soften scar tissue. Incorporating these creams into your post-surgical care routine can be a valuable addition to your anti-fibrosis therapeutic modalities.

LEARN MORE:

Scan or click here to learn about the best creams for fibrosis treatment.

89

WHAT IS THE BASIC TECHNIQUE FOR LYMPHATIC DRAINAGE SELF-MASSAGE AFTER 360 LIPOSUCTION?

After 360 liposuction, self-administered lymphatic drainage massage can be beneficial for promoting lymphatic flow and reducing swelling. Here's the basic technique you can try:

1. Start with Deep Breaths: Begin by taking a few deep breaths to relax your body and mind.

2. Lightly Warm the Area: You can use a warm compress or gently rub your hands together to create some warmth. This helps to improve circulation and makes the massage more effective.

3. Neck and Collarbone Strokes: Gently stroke your neck and collarbone area with your fingertips. Use light pressure and move your fingers in a gentle pumping motion towards the center of your collarbone.

4. Underarm Strokes: Place your hands under your arms and gently stroke upwards towards your armpits. This helps to stimulate the lymph nodes in the underarm area.

5. Stomach Strokes: Use gentle, circular motions with your fingertips to massage the stomach area. Start from the lower abdomen and move upwards towards the ribcage.

6. Hip Strokes: With your fingertips, stroke from the hip area towards the groin. This helps to stimulate lymphatic flow in the lower body.

7. Back Strokes: If possible, reach behind and gently stroke your lower back upwards towards the middle of your back. Use light pressure and repeat several times.

8. Thigh Strokes: Stroke the thighs in an upward direction towards the groin area. Use gentle pressure and repeat the motion several times.

Note:

Self-massage after 360 liposuction has some limitations that need to be considered. Given the large body areas involved, including the abdomen, flanks, and back, there is often a certain level of pain and discomfort after surgery, making self-massage challenging, especially during the early stages of recovery. Additionally, accessing the front of the stomach for manual massage may be manageable, but performing effective manual massage on the back is quite limited and may mostly rely on using massagers or other tools.

Moreover, managing such a large treatment area through self-massage can be physically demanding and may exceed what your body is ready for during the initial stages of recovery. Performing extensive self-massage on your own may not only be challenging but also tiring and potentially detrimental to your healing process.

To ensure a more effective and comfortable recovery after 360 liposuction, undergoing professional LM is highly recommended. Skilled LM therapists are trained to address specific post-operative needs and understand how to target the affected areas with precision and care. They can tailor their techniques to your unique condition and provide the appropriate level of pressure and strokes to enhance lymphatic drainage and reduce swelling.

Professional LM sessions not only facilitate quicker recovery in the immediate post-surgery period but also contribute to long-term benefits. Through regular sessions, LM can help prevent the development of fibrosis and support your body's natural healing process, leading to better overall outcomes in the long run.

Tip:

The good news is that LM after liposuction is one of the most utilized applications of Manual Lymphatic Drainage for postoperative recovery. Many experienced LM therapists are well-versed in the specific techniques required to address the needs of individuals recovering from body liposuction procedures.

Since liposuction can lead to swelling, bruising, and the potential development of fibrosis, LM plays a crucial role in expediting the healing process and promoting positive outcomes. The targeted strokes and gentle movements applied during LM help to redirect excess fluid away from the surgical areas, enhancing the body's natural ability to drain and eliminate it efficiently.

The popularity of LM after liposuction stems from its proven effectiveness in reducing postoperative edema, minimizing discomfort, and achieving smoother, more natural-looking results. Many patients experience faster recovery times and improved overall well-being with the incorporation of LM into their post-liposuction care plan.

LEARN MORE:

Scan or click here to watch video instructions for self-lymphatic massage after 360 liposuction.

90

WHAT IS THE BASIC TECHNIQUE FOR LYMPHATIC DRAINAGE SELF-MASSAGE AFTER ABDOMINOPLASTY?

Self-massage after abdominoplasty, also known as a tummy tuck, can be beneficial for promoting lymphatic drainage and reducing postoperative swelling.

1. Starting Position: Find a comfortable and relaxed position, such as lying on your back or sitting in a reclined position. Ensure your body is adequately supported and comfortable.

2. Deep Breathing: Begin with a few deep breaths to relax your body and mind. Deep breathing can also aid in promoting lymphatic flow.

3. Gentle Strokes: Using light pressure, gently stroke the skin on your abdomen with your fingertips or palms. Start from the center of your abdomen (around the navel area) and stroke outward towards your sides.

4. Circular Motion: Using your fingertips, make gentle circular motions around the incision area and the surrounding tissues. Gradually move in larger circles to encompass the entire abdomen.

5. Upward Strokes: From your lower abdomen, stroke upward towards your ribcage. This motion helps direct fluid towards the upper body's lymphatic drainage pathways.

6. Lateral Strokes: Stroke from the midline of your abdomen towards your sides, following the natural lymphatic flow. This technique encourages fluid drainage towards the inguinal (groin) lymph nodes.

7. Repeat: Continue these gentle strokes for about five to ten minutes, ensuring that you apply minimal pressure, especially over the incision area.

8. Frequency: You can perform self-massage several times a day, as recommended by your surgeon or LM therapist. Start self-massage only after getting approval from your surgeon during follow-up visits.

Note:

The self LM technique for the front of the abdomen after abdominoplasty is different due to the presence of a lower transverse abdominal incision. This incision completely disrupts the lymphatic communication between the skin and soft tissue above and below the incision. As a result, fluid from above the incision is no longer able to be transferred naturally to the groin lymphatic collectors.

However, the skin and soft tissue below the incision still preserve their connection to the groin lymphatic collection, and fluid transition in this area is not disrupted. Massage in this area should be directed towards the groin lymph nodes to facilitate fluid drainage.

Fluid from the areas above the incision line needs to be directed via accessory lymphatic pathways located on the flanks. These accessory pathways are not as developed as the main ones and can transit a smaller volume of fluid. Additionally, the transit of edema fluid via these accessory pathways is hindered by gravitational forces, which further complicates the elimination of excessive fluid from the area above the lower abdominal incision line.

Tip:

Above the abdominal scar, perform slow, gentle strokes away from the lower incision site towards the sides, extending more superiorly to the sides of the body.

Below the incision, apply the same type of strokes toward the groin lymphatic collector areas located in the right and left groin creases.

Always ensure that the pressure is light and comfortable during the massage. Perform this technique with caution, especially around the incision area, and follow any specific instructions provided by your surgeon or LM therapist.

LEARN MORE:

Scan or click here to watch video instructions for self-lymphatic massage after abdominoplasty.

91

WHAT IS THE BASIC TECHNIQUE FOR LYMPHATIC DRAINAGE SELF-MASSAGE AFTER BREAST REDUCTION OR LIFT?

Basic Technique for Lymphatic Drainage Self Massage after Breast Reduction or Lift:

1. Start by finding a comfortable and relaxed position, either sitting or lying down, with your back and shoulders well-supported.

2. Gently place your hands on your breasts, ensuring a light touch and using your fingertips to avoid applying excessive pressure.

3. Perform slow, rhythmic strokes with your hands, moving in gentle circular motions towards the outer areas of your breasts. This movement should be in the direction of the lymphatic flow, which is towards the armpits and upper chest.

4. Continue the circular strokes, gradually working your way up towards your armpits and the upper chest. This helps to facilitate the drainage of lymphatic fluid towards the lymph nodes in these areas.

5. After completing the circular strokes, use soft pumping motions with your hands over the breast tissue. This helps to further encourage lymphatic flow and drainage.

6. Next, gently sweep your hands from the center of your chest outwards, towards the sides of your body. Repeat this movement multiple times.

7. Pay attention to any areas of tenderness or tightness, and spend extra time massaging those areas with gentle strokes.

Note:

Remember to breathe deeply and relax during the self-massage to maximize its effectiveness. Perform this self-massage regularly, following the guidance of your healthcare provider, to promote lymphatic drainage and reduce swelling and discomfort after breast reduction or lift surgery.

Tip:

Compression post-surgical bras play a vital role in reducing swelling and providing support after breast surgery. Typically, your surgeon will provide you with a post-surgical bra to wear during the initial recovery period. However, it is essential to ensure that the bra fits comfortably and does not cause excessive pressure or irritation to the skin.

While wearing a surgical bra is widely recommended, each individual's body is different, and some may find that the provided bra may not be the most suitable option for them. If you experience any discomfort or find the provided bra to be too tight, it is crucial to communicate this with your surgeon or LM specialist.

The right fit and comfort of the surgical bra are paramount for your recovery. Look for a bra that offers adequate support without being overly restrictive. Opt for one made of soft, breathable materials that will not cause irritation or chafing. Some surgical bras also have adjustable straps or bands, allowing you to customize the fit to your specific needs.

As soon as you are cleared by your surgeon to switch to a different type of bra, consider trying out different options to find the one that works best for you. Many brands offer specialized post-surgical bras designed for optimal comfort and support during recovery.

Remember, proper support and comfort are essential during the healing process. By choosing the right compression post-surgical bra, you can ensure that you are providing your body with the best conditions for a smooth and successful recovery after breast surgery.

LEARN MORE:

Scan or click here to find more tips on finding a perfect post-surgical bra.

92

WHAT IS THE BASIC TECHNIQUE FOR LYMPHATIC DRAINAGE SELF-MASSAGE AFTER A FACE LIFT?

Basic Technique for Lymphatic Drainage Self Massage after a Face Lift:

1. Begin by finding a comfortable and relaxed position, either sitting or lying down, with your head and neck well-supported.

2. Gently place your hands on your face, using a light touch and your fingertips for the massage.

3. Start by performing slow, gentle strokes from the center of your face outwards, towards your temples. These strokes should follow the natural direction of lymphatic flow in the face.

4. Continue with circular motions, working your way around your cheeks and jawline. Remember to keep the pressure light and avoid pulling on the skin.

5. Next, focus on the area around your ears and neck, as lymph nodes are located in these regions. Use soft pumping motions with your fingertips to encourage lymphatic drainage.

6. Pay special attention to any areas of swelling or tenderness, and spend extra time massaging those areas with gentle strokes.

7. After completing the face massage, move on to the neck and perform slow, rhythmic strokes from the bottom of your neck upwards towards your chin.

8. Throughout the massage, remember to breathe deeply and try to relax your facial muscles.

9. Perform this self-massage regularly, as advised by your surgeon or LM therapist, to help reduce swelling, promote healing, and enhance the overall recovery process after your face lift surgery.

Note:

A face lift is an invasive procedure that involves the manipulation and alteration of delicate facial and neck tissues, which can disrupt the complex system of lymphatic drainage in these areas. To ensure effective and safe self-LM after a face lift, it is highly recommended to learn appropriate techniques from your LM therapist and practice them under their supervision initially.

Tip:

Performing LM after a face lift in front of a mirror allows for more precise localization of pressure areas and direction of massage strokes. By observing yourself in the mirror, you can better understand the contours of your face, identify areas of swelling or tenderness, and tailor the massage technique accordingly.

LEARN MORE:

Scan or click <u>here</u> to learn more about recovery after a face lift.

23

WHAT IS THE BASIC TECHNIQUE FOR LYMPHATIC DRAINAGE SELF-MASSAGE AFTER BLEPHAROPLASTY?

After blepharoplasty, it is essential to be gentle and cautious while performing self-lymphatic drainage (LM) around the delicate eye area. Here is the basic technique for self LM after blepharoplasty:

1. Clean Hands: Before starting the self LM, ensure that your hands are clean to avoid any risk of infection.

2. Gently Tapping and Pulsing: With your fingertips, perform gentle tapping or pulsing motions on the areas surrounding the eyes. Start from the inner corners of the eyes and move outwards towards the temples. Avoid direct pressure on the eyelids or any incision sites.

3. Circular Massage: Using light pressure, perform small circular motions with your fingertips on the bony area around the eyes. Move in a clockwise direction, starting from the inner corner of the eye and working your way outwards.

4. Lymphatic Flow Direction: Always keep the natural lymphatic flow direction in mind. Encourage fluid movement towards the lymph nodes located near the temples and sides of the neck.

5. Eyebrow Strokes: Place your fingertips at the inner corner of the eyebrows and gently stroke outwards towards the temples. This can help to facilitate lymphatic drainage in the area.

6. Relaxation Techniques: You can incorporate relaxation techniques like deep breathing during the self LM to help reduce tension and promote overall relaxation.

7. Duration and Frequency: Perform self LM for a few minutes at a time, two to three times a day, to help improve lymphatic circulation and reduce post-operative swelling.

8. Be Mindful: Make a mental note of any discomfort or pain during the self LM. If you experience any discomfort, stop the massage immediately and consult with your surgeon or healthcare provider.

Note:

Remember, the area around the eyes is sensitive, and after blepharoplasty, it may be even more delicate. Always follow the specific post-surgery instructions provided by your surgeon and consult with your healthcare team before starting self LM to ensure that it is appropriate for your individual case.

After certain surgical procedures, such as blepharoplasty or eyelid surgery, it is common for surgeons to recommend the use of antibiotic ointments to prevent infection and promote healing. When discussing your post-operative care with your surgeon, inquire about the possibility of using safe antibiotic ointments that can also be used for LM. If your surgeon approves the use of such ointments, they can serve a dual purpose by facilitating the healing process and also assisting in LM.

Tip:

A regular Q-Tip, commonly used for various applications in medicine and skincare, can serve a dual purpose in your post-operative care after eyelid surgery. Apart from its use in applying antibiotic ointment to the sutured area to promote healing, it can also be utilized as an excellent tool for lymphatic drainage (LM) in the delicate eyelid region.

The soft and cotton-tipped end of a Q-Tip allows for gentle and precise strokes, making it ideal for performing LM in the small and sensitive areas of the eyelids. By gently gliding the Q-Tip along the eyelid contours, you can promote the circulation of lymphatic fluid and reduce any post-operative swelling or bruising effectively.

Using a Q-Tip for lymphatic drainage ensures that the massage is performed with care and minimal pressure, which is crucial for the tender eyelid skin. This technique can aid in the reduction of puffiness and promote the body's natural healing process.

However, it is essential to approach self-massage with a Q-Tip cautiously and under the guidance of your surgeon or LM therapist. They can provide you with specific instructions on the correct technique and frequency of self-massage, ensuring that you are using the Q-Tip safely and effectively.

By combining the application of antibiotic ointment and lymphatic drainage with a Q-Tip, you can support your post-operative recovery and enhance the healing process in the sensitive areas around the eyes. Always follow the recommendations of your healthcare professionals to ensure a smooth and successful recovery after your eyelid surgery.

LEARN MORE:

Scan or click here to learn more about recovery after eyelid surgery.

94

WHICH ESSENTIAL OILS ARE BENEFICIAL FOR LYMPHATIC DRAINAGE?

Several essential oils have been known to support lymphatic drainage and promote a healthy lymphatic system. Here are some essential oils that can be helpful:

1. **Lemon Essential Oil:** This oil is known for its detoxifying properties and can support lymphatic drainage by promoting fluid circulation and helping to flush out toxins.

2. **Grapefruit Essential Oil:** This fruit is a natural diuretic and can help reduce water retention, making it beneficial for lymphatic drainage.

3. **Cypress Essential Oil:** It has astringent properties that can support lymphatic flow and reduce swelling.

4. **Ginger Essential Oil:** This oil has anti-inflammatory properties that can help reduce inflammation in the lymphatic system and improve circulation.

5. **Rosemary Essential Oil:** This can support lymphatic drainage by improving blood flow and reducing swelling.

6. **Helichrysum Essential Oil:** It is known for its anti-inflammatory and regenerative properties, making it beneficial for promoting lymphatic health.

Note:

When using essential oils for lymphatic drainage, it's essential to dilute them properly in a carrier oil before applying them topically. Always ensure you are using pure, high-quality essential oils from reputable sources, as synthetic or low-quality oils may not provide the same benefits. It's also a good idea to consult with a qualified aromatherapist or healthcare professional to determine the best essential oil blends and usage for your specific needs.

Tip:

Essential oils are potent and should never be applied directly to the skin, as they can cause irritation. It is essential to dilute them properly in base oils, such as coconut or hemp seed oil before use. Professional LM therapists typically use high-quality oils during their MLD sessions to ensure safety and effectiveness. If you prefer not to mix essential oils for lymphatic drainage at home, it is advisable to look for commercially available pre-mixed blends that are specifically designed for this purpose. These blends are carefully formulated to support lymphatic flow and can be added to carrier oils or body lotions for self-massage. By incorporating these blends into your massage routine, you can enhance the benefits of lymphatic drainage and promote overall well-being.

LEARN MORE:

Scan or click <u>here</u> to learn more about essential oils that are beneficial for lymphatic drainage.

95

IS THERE ANY SPECIFIC SKINCARE NEEDED FOR THE AREA OF LIPOSUCTION?

Yes, there are some specific skincare considerations for the area of liposuction. After the procedure, it is essential to keep the treated skin clean and dry to prevent infection and promote healing. Your surgeon may provide specific instructions on how to care for the incision sites and manage any dressings or bandages.

Additionally, it's crucial to avoid exposing the treated areas to direct sunlight or tanning beds during the initial healing phase, as this can lead to hyperpigmentation or other skin issues. Applying a broad-spectrum sunscreen to the treated areas when going outside is recommended.

You may also be advised to use a mild and gentle cleanser for the first few days after the surgery to avoid irritating the skin. As the healing progresses, your surgeon may recommend using moisturizers or scar creams to help improve the appearance of any scars and keep the skin hydrated.

Note:

LM has numerous benefits, not only for deep soft tissue recovery but also for skin recovery. By aiding in the elimination of excessive fluid and promoting gentle stretching of the skin, LM can accelerate the healing process of vital skin components like collagen and elastic fibers. Consequently, the skin regains its tone and experiences improved laxity, leading to a more youthful appearance.

In conjunction with MLD, the use of specific topical skincare products can further enhance skin regeneration during the recovery period. Lymphedema specialists stress the importance of selecting products with a neutral pH for individuals with lymphedema. The skin in such cases can be sensitive to variations in the acidity of topical creams and lotions, making it essential to opt for products with a neutral pH to maintain skin health and minimize potential irritations.

By incorporating both LM and appropriate skincare products with neutral pH levels into your postoperative care routine, you can maximize the benefits of the treatments and foster a more efficient and satisfying recovery process for both deep tissues and the skin. Always consult with your healthcare professional or LM therapist to ensure the products you use align with your specific needs and promote optimal healing.

Tip:

Before applying any new topical skincare product to the recovering areas after surgery, it is crucial to conduct a patch test. Begin by trying the product on a small, untreated part of your body to ensure that there are no allergic reactions or adverse effects to the ingredients. This precautionary step is essential to prevent any potential complications or irritations on the sensitive postoperative skin.

Once you have confirmed that the product is safe and well-tolerated on the test area, you can confidently apply it to the areas where you are recovering from surgery. Take care to follow the recommended application guidelines and be gentle while massaging the product into the skin. A smooth and even application can help maximize the product's benefits without causing unnecessary stress on the healing tissues.

LEARN MORE:

Scan or click here for more tips on skincare after plastic surgery.

96

WHAT IS KINESIOLOGY TAPE?

Kinesiology tape, often referred to as kinesio tape or KT tape, is a special type of flexible adhesive tape used for therapeutic purposes in sports and rehabilitation settings. It was developed in the 1970s by Japanese chiropractor Dr. Kenzo Kase.

The tape is made of cotton fibers with an acrylic adhesive on one side, designed to mimic the elasticity and thickness of human skin. This unique composition allows the tape to stretch longitudinally, providing support and stability to muscles and joints without restricting movement. The adhesive is hypoallergenic and latex-free, making it suitable for most individuals, including those with sensitive skin.

Kinesiology tape is commonly used to support injured or strained muscles, reduce pain, improve circulation, and promote lymphatic drainage. It is believed to provide proprioceptive feedback to the body, which may help improve muscle activation and overall performance during physical activities.

The application of kinesiology tape is specific to each individual's needs and the targeted area of treatment. It is commonly used by athletes, physical therapists, and other healthcare professionals to manage various musculoskeletal conditions and aid in the recovery process.

Note:

Kinesiology tape has gained popularity as an adjunct to LM due to its potential benefits in promoting lymphatic drainage in the treated area. When applied properly, the tape can provide a gentle lifting and stretching effect on the skin, which can help facilitate the movement of lymphatic fluid through the lymphatic vessels.

The benefits of using kinesiology tape for lymphatic drainage include:

1. **Improved Lymphatic Flow:** The lifting effect of the tape can create extra space between the skin and the underlying tissues, allowing lymphatic fluid to flow more freely. This can help reduce swelling and edema in the treated area.

2. **Enhanced Circulation:** The tape's unique elastic properties can stimulate blood circulation, which in turn can support the removal of waste products and toxins from the affected area.

3. **Reduced Pain and Discomfort:** Kinesiology tape can provide gentle support to muscles and joints, which may help alleviate pain and discomfort associated with lymphatic congestion.

4. **Extended Benefits:** Unlike traditional bandages or compression garments, kinesiology tape is flexible and can be worn for several days, providing ongoing support and lymphatic drainage even after the LM session is completed.

5. **Comfort and Versatility:** Kinesiology tape is lightweight and breathable, offering comfort to the wearer. It can be applied to various body parts and can adapt to different

shapes and movements, making it suitable for various applications.

When used in conjunction with LM, kinesiology tape can complement the effects of the massage and help maintain the benefits of increased lymphatic drainage for a longer period. However, it is essential to ensure proper application by a qualified LM therapist or healthcare professional to achieve optimal results and avoid any adverse effects.

Tip:

Before applying kinesiology tape over the body areas after liposuction, it's essential to ensure that the skin is clean, dry, and free from any oils or lotions. Follow these step-by-step instructions for proper application:

1. **Measure and Cut:** Using a pair of scissors, cut the kinesiology tape to the desired length, allowing enough tape to cover the target area.

2. **Rounded Corners:** To prevent the tape from peeling prematurely, round the corners of the tape before application.

3. **Prepare the Skin:** Gently clean the skin with mild soap and water, and pat it dry. Avoid using any lotions or oils on the area.

4. **Apply the Tape:** Start by gently stretching the kinesiology tape. Apply the middle part of the tape directly over the targeted area, ensuring that it is aligned with the surrounding skin.

5. **Smooth the Tape:** Use light pressure to smooth the tape down onto the skin. Be careful not to stretch the tape excessively, as this can cause discomfort or skin irritation.

6. **Create Tension:** For lymphatic drainage purposes, gently stretch the ends of the tape without applying too much tension. This creates a lifting effect on the skin, which can facilitate lymphatic fluid flow.

7. **Round off the Edges:** To ensure that the edges of the tape do not peel off, rub the entire surface of the tape with your palm to activate the adhesive.

8. **Avoid Wrinkles:** Check for any wrinkles or folds in the tape and smooth them out gently.

9. **Movement and Breathability:** Kinesiology tape is designed to move with the body and allow the skin to breathe. Make sure the tape is comfortable and does not restrict movement.

10. **Observe Sensations:** After applying the tape, pay attention to any sensations or discomfort. If the tape feels too tight or causes irritation, remove it immediately and consult your LM therapist or healthcare provider.

Remember that kinesiology tape should only be applied by a qualified LM therapist or under their guidance. Improper application may not provide the desired benefits and can lead to adverse effects. Additionally, kinesiology tape should not be applied over open wounds or damaged skin.

LEARN MORE:

Scan or click here to learn about benefits of kinesiology tape in scar care.

97

WHAT IS WOOD (OR WOODEN) THERAPY FOR POSTOPERATIVE RECOVERY?

Wood (or wooden) therapy, also known as maderotherapy, is a manual massage technique that involves the use of specially designed wooden tools to perform massage and body contouring. It has gained popularity as a postoperative recovery treatment in combination with lymphatic drainage massage for cosmetic surgery patients.

During the wood therapy session, the therapist uses various wooden tools in different shapes and sizes to apply pressure, friction, and rolling movements to the body's soft tissues. These tools are typically made of high-quality hardwood and are carefully crafted to target specific areas of the body.

For postoperative recovery, wood therapy is often used in conjunction with lymphatic drainage massage to help reduce swelling, inflammation, and bruising after cosmetic surgery procedures like liposuction, tummy tucks, or Brazilian butt lifts. The gentle yet effective massage techniques of wood therapy can aid in promoting lymphatic circulation, encouraging the removal of excess fluids and toxins from the body, and speeding up the healing process.

Note:

The pressure and movements applied during wood therapy can also help to break down fibrous tissue and promote collagen production, resulting in improved skin texture and tone. Additionally, the massage helps to relax the muscles, relieve tension, and provide a sense of overall well-being, which can be particularly beneficial for patients during the postoperative recovery period.

Tip:

Wood therapy, as part of postoperative massage, should be performed carefully to avoid discomfort and pain. It involves the use of various wooden tools specially designed to provide specific massage benefits. The selection of the right wooden tool is essential to ensure a safe and effective treatment.

There are several variations of wooden massagers used in wood therapy, each serving a unique purpose. Some tools are designed for deep tissue massage to target specific areas of tension and fibrosis, promoting circulation and reducing postoperative swelling. Other tools are used for gentle lymphatic drainage massage, encouraging the removal of excess fluid and toxins from the body.

LEARN MORE:

Scan or click here to learn more about benefits of wooden therapy for recovery after plastic surgery.

98

WHAT CONSUMABLE PRODUCTS CAN HELP TO ENHANCE LYMPHATIC DRAINAGE?

There are numerous products available in different forms to support and enhance natural body lymphatic drainage. Here are some common types of products that can aid in promoting a healthy lymphatic system:

1. **Supplements in Capsule or Tablet Form:** Lymphatic drainage supplements often come in the form of capsules or tablets containing a combination of herbs, vitamins, and minerals known for their lymphatic-supporting properties. These supplements may include ingredients such as dandelion root, red clover, cleavers, and vitamin C, among others.

2. **Lymphatic Drainage Tinctures (Drops):** Tinctures are liquid herbal extracts that can be taken orally or added to water or juice. Lymphatic drainage tinctures typically contain concentrated herbal extracts with lymphatic-

stimulating properties. They are easy to use and allow for customizable dosages.

3. **Lymphatic Drainage Tea:** These teas are herbal blends specifically formulated to promote healthy lymphatic function. They often include ingredients like ginger, turmeric, burdock root, and licorice, which have anti-inflammatory and diuretic properties to support lymph flow.

4. **Lymphatic Drainage Super Greens Powder:** These are nutrient-dense blends of green vegetables, algae, and other plant-based ingredients. Some super greens formulations also include herbs that support lymphatic flow, making them a convenient way to boost overall nutrition and support the lymphatic system.

5. **Lymphatic Drainage Shots:** These are concentrated liquid supplements that are designed to be taken in small doses. These shots may contain a combination of herbs, vitamins, and minerals that are beneficial for lymphatic health. They provide a quick and efficient way to deliver essential nutrients to support lymphatic drainage.

Note:

It's important to note that while these products can be helpful, they are not a substitute for overall healthy lifestyle habits, such as a balanced diet, regular exercise, proper hydration, and adequate rest. Additionally, individual responses to these products may vary, and it's always best to consult with a healthcare professional before starting any new supplements, especially if you have existing health conditions or are taking medications. Integrating these products as part of a comprehensive approach to lymphatic health can be beneficial in supporting your body's natural detoxification and immune processes.

Tip:

Most consumable products designed to promote lymphatic drainage often contain similar key ingredients known for their beneficial effects on the lymphatic system. These ingredients may include herbal extracts like dandelion root, burdock, red clover, ginger, and turmeric, as well as vitamins and minerals such as vitamin C and potassium.

To make the selection process easier, consider the type of product that best suits your preferences and lifestyle. For example, if you prefer the convenience of capsules or tablets, look for a high-quality lymphatic drainage supplement in that form. On the other hand, if you enjoy the ritual of sipping on soothing beverages, a lymphatic drainage tea may be the perfect choice for you.

It's essential to stick to one specific product and not consume multiple products with similar ingredients simultaneously. Taking multiple products with overlapping ingredients may lead to excessive intake of certain compounds, which could potentially be harmful or result in unwanted side effects. By choosing one well-rounded lymphatic drainage product that aligns with your preferences, you can ensure a balanced intake of the necessary nutrients and support your lymphatic system effectively.

Additionally, if you have any existing health conditions or are taking medications, consult with a healthcare professional before adding any new supplements to your regimen. They can help you determine the appropriate dosage and ensure that the product is safe and suitable for your individual needs.

LEARN MORE:

Scan or click <u>here</u> to learn more about benefits of lymphatic drainage bath salts.

99

WHAT HERBAL TEAS ARE BENEFICIAL FOR LYMPHATIC DRAINAGE AFTER SURGERY?

Several herbal teas are known for their potential benefits in supporting lymphatic drainage and promoting post-surgery recovery. Some of the beneficial herbal teas include:

1. **Dandelion Root Tea:** This root is believed to have diuretic properties that may help reduce water retention and promote lymphatic flow.

2. **Burdock Root Tea:** This root is known for its detoxifying properties and is believed to support lymphatic drainage.

3. **Red Clover Tea:** This is thought to help cleanse the lymphatic system and improve lymphatic circulation.

4. **Ginger Tea:** It has anti-inflammatory properties that may aid in reducing swelling and promoting lymphatic flow.

5. **Turmeric Tea:** This contains curcumin, a powerful antioxidant with anti-inflammatory effects that may support lymphatic function.

6. **Nettle Tea:** This is believed to have diuretic properties, which may assist in flushing out excess fluid from the body.

7. **Cleavers Tea:** It is traditionally used to support the lymphatic system and aid in detoxification.

8. **Fennel Tea:** It may help improve digestion, which can indirectly support lymphatic drainage.

9. **Green Tea:** This is rich in antioxidants and may aid in reducing inflammation and supporting the lymphatic system.

10. **Chamomile Tea:** It has anti-inflammatory properties and may help promote relaxation, which can be beneficial for lymphatic drainage.

Note:

When choosing herbal teas for lymphatic drainage, opt for high-quality organic teas whenever possible to ensure you're getting the full benefits of the herbs. It's essential to consult with your healthcare provider, especially if you have any medical conditions or are taking medications, as some herbal teas may interact with certain medications or have contraindications.

Tip:

Commercially available tea blends specifically formulated for lymphatic drainage can indeed offer a convenient and effective way to support your body's natural detoxification processes, both for regular use and postoperative recovery. These blends typically contain a combination of key ingredients known for their lymphatic health benefits, making them more potent and targeted than single herbal teas.

These carefully blended teas are often formulated to taste pleasant and can be enjoyed as part of a daily wellness routine or incorporated into your postoperative recovery plan to assist in reducing swelling and promoting healing. Always choose reputable brands with high-quality organic ingredients to ensure the tea's effectiveness and safety.

It's essential to follow the recommended dosage and consult with your healthcare provider before incorporating any new herbal teas or supplements into your routine, especially if you have any health conditions or are taking medications.

LEARN MORE:

Scan or click here to learn how to make lymphatic tea at home.

100

DOES ARNICA TEA HELP WITH LYMPHATIC DRAINAGE?

Arnica is an herb known for its anti-inflammatory properties and is commonly used in various forms to promote healing and reduce swelling and bruising. While Arnica has been used topically as a cream or ointment for bruises and muscle soreness, there is limited evidence to support the use of Arnica tea specifically for lymphatic drainage.

Arnica tea is not as commonly used as topical Arnica preparations, and its effectiveness for lymphatic drainage has not been extensively studied. The active compounds in Arnica, such as sesquiterpene lactones, are more concentrated in topical preparations rather than teas.

Note:

For promoting lymphatic drainage, other herbal teas like those containing dandelion root, burdock root, red clover, ginger, turmeric, and nettle are more commonly recommended due to their well-documented diuretic, anti-inflammatory, and lymphatic-supportive properties.

Tip:

Yes, Arnica Montana is considered toxic when taken orally. It contains compounds known as sesquiterpene lactones, which can be harmful if ingested in large amounts. Consuming Arnica Montana orally can lead to various adverse effects, including nausea, vomiting, abdominal pain, dizziness, and in severe cases, it can even be life-threatening.

Due to its potential toxicity, Arnica montana should never be ingested as a tea or any other form of oral intake unless it is in highly diluted homeopathic preparations, which are specially formulated to be safe for oral use. Even in homeopathic preparations, it is essential to follow the recommended dosages and guidelines provided by a qualified homeopathic practitioner.

To ensure your safety, it is best to use Arnica Montana topically, in the form of creams, ointments, or gels, or in homeopathic preparations specifically designed for external use. Always consult with a healthcare professional or a qualified herbalist before using Arnica montana or any other herbal remedy, especially if you are pregnant, breastfeeding, or have any medical conditions or allergies.

LEARN MORE:

Scan or click here to learn about safe use of Arnica products.

BONUS QUESTIONS:

101

WHAT IS THE APPROPRIATE AMOUNT OF HYDRATION BEFORE AND AFTER LYMPHATIC MASSAGE SESSION?

The recommendation for hydration before and after an LM session is to stay well-hydrated. It is essential to drink plenty of water throughout the day, both before and after the session. Adequate hydration helps optimize the effects of the massage and supports the body's lymphatic system in eliminating waste and toxins. Keeping the body well-hydrated also aids in reducing post-massage soreness and promotes overall well-being.

Aim to consume water at regular intervals, and don't wait until you feel parched. Keeping a water bottle handy and sipping water frequently can help you maintain proper hydration levels. Staying ahead of your body's hydration needs allows the lymphatic system to function efficiently, facilitating the removal of waste and toxins from the body.

Note:

During and after the LM session, it is equally important to continue hydrating. Hydration supports the body in flushing out any toxins that may have been released during the massage. Drinking water post-session can also help alleviate any potential soreness or discomfort that could occur because of the massage.

Incorporate other hydrating beverages, such as herbal teas or electrolyte-enhanced drinks, to add variety to your hydration routine. Remember, staying consistently hydrated is a proactive step in supporting your body's natural functions and optimizing the benefits of LM for your overall well-being.

Tip:

Doubling your usual volume of liquids consumed during the days you have a professional LM session is a beneficial practice to ensure proper hydration and maximize the benefits of the massage. Hydration is a key factor in supporting the lymphatic system's efficiency and promoting the elimination of waste and toxins from the body.

When preparing for a professional LM session, focus on increasing your water intake significantly. This includes not only drinking water but also incorporating other hydrating beverages such as herbal teas, fresh fruit juices, and electrolyte-rich drinks.

Start increasing your fluid intake at least a day before the scheduled LM session, and continue the practice on the day of the massage. Adequate hydration helps to optimize the circulation of lymphatic fluid and supports the body's natural detoxification processes.

LEARN MORE:

Scan or click <u>here</u> to learn about benefits of limiting dietary salt intake during recovery after plastic surgery.

102

HOW TO REDUCE DISCOMFORT DURING LYMPHATIC MASSAGE THERAPY?

To minimize pain during LM, you can follow these helpful tips:

1. **Communicate with your therapist:** Inform your LM therapist about your pain tolerance and any sensitive areas before the session. They can adjust their technique and pressure accordingly to ensure a more comfortable experience.

2. **Start gently:** If you're new to LM therapy or have areas of tenderness, ask your therapist to being with gentle strokes, and gradually increase pressure as you become more accustomed to the massage.

3. **Deep breathing:** Practice deep breathing during the session to help relax your body and reduce muscle tension. Deep breaths can also distract you from any discomfort.

4. **Warm up:** Apply a warm compress or take a warm shower before the session. Heat can help loosen up muscles and improve blood flow, making the massage more comfortable.

5. **Use pain-relieving creams or oils:** Topical pain-relieving products containing ingredients like arnica, menthol, or CBD can be applied before the massage to alleviate discomfort.

6. **Take breaks:** If you experience discomfort during the session, don't hesitate to ask your therapist for a short break to allow your body to relax.

7. **Stay hydrated:** Ensure you're well-hydrated before and after the session, as dehydration can worsen muscle tension and sensitivity.

8. **Relaxation techniques:** Practice relaxation techniques like visualization, meditation, or focusing on calming thoughts during the massage to divert your attention from any pain.

9. **Post-session care:** After the LM therapy, follow any post-massage instructions provided by your therapist. This may include using ice packs on sore areas, gentle stretching, or avoiding strenuous activities.

Note:

Choose a skilled therapist: Ensure you're working with a qualified and experienced LM therapist who understands your needs and can adjust the massage technique accordingly.

Always remember that some level of discomfort may be normal during certain parts of the LM therapy, especially if there's significant swelling or inflammation.

Tip:

It's essential to have a conversation with your LM therapist before your first session to discuss ways to reduce discomfort during the treatment. Mention any concerns you have about pain or sensitivity in certain areas so that the therapist can tailor the massage to your needs.

It's important to avoid taking narcotic-based pain medication before the LM session. These medications can cause side effects such as nausea, which may be exacerbated during the massage, especially if your body is undergoing detoxification. Instead, opt for more natural ways to manage discomfort, such as applying warm compresses, using topical pain-relieving creams, or practicing relaxation techniques.

LEARN MORE:

Scan or click here to learn more about additional ways to promote recovery after plastic surgery.

103

WHAT DIET BENEFITS LYMPHATIC DRAINAGE?

A diet that benefits lymphatic drainage is one that promotes overall health, reduces inflammation, and supports proper lymphatic function. Here are some dietary guidelines that can be beneficial for lymphatic drainage:

1. **Hydration:** Stay well-hydrated by drinking plenty of water throughout the day. Proper hydration helps to maintain lymphatic fluid flow and aids in the removal of waste and toxins from the body.

2. **Whole Foods:** Focus on a diet rich in whole, unprocessed foods such as fruits, vegetables, whole grains, lean proteins, and healthy fats. These foods provide essential nutrients and antioxidants that support lymphatic health and reduce inflammation.

3. **Reduce Salt Intake:** High salt intake can lead to water retention and swelling, which can impede lymphatic flow.

Limiting your salt intake can help to minimize water retention and support proper drainage.

4. **Limit Processed Foods:** These foods often contain unhealthy fats, excess salt, and additives that can contribute to inflammation and hinder lymphatic function. Aim to minimize processed foods in your diet.

5. **Healthy Fats:** Incorporate sources of healthy fats such as avocados, nuts, seeds, and olive oil. Healthy fats are important for cell function and support the absorption of fat-soluble vitamins.

6. **Fiber:** Include plenty of fiber in your diet from fruits, vegetables, and whole grains. Fiber aids in proper digestion and can help prevent constipation, which may contribute to lymphatic congestion.

7. **Herbal Teas:** Some herbal teas, such as dandelion tea, ginger tea, and green tea, have been associated with supporting lymphatic function. These teas can be included as part of a balanced diet.

8. **Manage Alcohol and Caffeine:** Limiting alcohol and caffeine intake can help reduce dehydration and support better lymphatic fluid flow.

Note:

Preparing for challenges with nutrition after a plastic surgery procedure is essential to support the healing process and overall recovery. Here are some practical tips to help you:

1. **Plan Meals in Advance:** Before your surgery, create a meal plan that includes nutrient-dense foods and easy-to-prepare options. Consider preparing some meals in advance and freezing them for easy access during your recovery.

2. **Stock up on Healthy Snacks:** Have a variety of healthy snacks readily available, such as cut-up fruits, nuts, yogurt, or whole-grain crackers. These snacks can be convenient during times when you may not have the energy to cook a full meal.

3. **Include Protein in Your Diet:** Protein is essential for tissue repair and healing. Incorporate lean protein sources such as chicken, fish, tofu, beans, and lentils into your meals.

6. **Consider Supplements:** Consult with your surgeon or a registered dietitian about whether certain supplements, like vitamin C or zinc, may be beneficial for your recovery.

7. **Be Mindful of Dietary Restrictions:** If you have any dietary restrictions or allergies, ensure that you communicate these with your caregivers and have appropriate alternatives available.

8. **Listen to Your Body:** Pay attention to your body's cues and eat when you feel hungry. Don't force yourself to eat large meals if you're not feeling up to it; instead, opt for smaller, frequent meals.

9. **Follow Your Surgeon's Guidelines:** Always follow your surgeon's post-operative dietary guidelines. They may have specific recommendations based on the procedure and your individual health needs.

Tip:

Here is a list of foods that are considered beneficial for lymphatic drainage:

1. **Fruits:** Berries (blueberries, strawberries, raspberries), oranges, lemons, limes, grapefruit, kiwi, pineapple, watermelon, and papaya.

2. **Vegetables:** Leafy greens (spinach, kale, Swiss chard), broccoli, cauliflower, Brussels sprouts, cabbage, asparagus, beets, carrots, and celery.

3. **Herbs and Spices:** Turmeric, ginger, garlic, cilantro, parsley, and dandelion.

4. **Healthy Fats:** Avocado, nuts (almonds, walnuts), seeds (chia seeds, flaxseeds), and extra virgin olive oil.

5. **Whole Grains:** Brown rice, quinoa, oats, and barley.

6. **Lean Proteins:** Fish (salmon, trout), chicken, turkey, tofu, and legumes (beans, lentils).

7. **Herbal Teas:** Dandelion tea, ginger tea, green tea, and chamomile tea.

8. **Healthy Fluids:** Water, coconut water, and herbal-infused water.

9. **Probiotic Foods:** Yogurt (unsweetened and probiotic-rich), kefir, sauerkraut, and kimchi.

10. **Dark Chocolate:** In moderation, dark chocolate (70% or higher cocoa content) contains antioxidants that may be beneficial.

Remember, the overall focus should be on maintaining a well-balanced diet with plenty of whole, unprocessed foods, as well as staying well-hydrated. Including these foods as part of a healthy lifestyle can support lymphatic drainage and overall well-being. It's always best to consult with a healthcare professional or registered dietitian for personalized dietary advice based on individual health needs and goals.

LEARN MORE:

Scan or click <u>here</u> for recipes for the top three lymphatic drainage smoothies.

104

WHAT IS A FAJA?

A faja is a type of compression garment commonly used after various surgical procedures, including liposuction, tummy tuck (abdominoplasty), and other body contouring surgeries. It is a form-fitting garment made from elastic and/or compression fabrics that provides support and compression to the treated areas.

The primary purpose of wearing a faja is to help control swelling, reduce fluid buildup, and promote proper healing in the postoperative period. The compression provided by the faja helps to shape and contour the body, ensuring that the skin adheres to the underlying tissues, reducing the risk of sagging or loose skin after surgery.

Fajas come in different styles and designs to fit various body shapes and surgical needs. Some fajas cover specific areas, such as the abdomen or thighs, while others may provide full-body coverage. They may have different levels of compression and be adjustable to accommodate changes in swelling and body shape during the recovery process.

Wearing a faja is an essential part of the postoperative care plan, as it helps improve blood circulation and lymphatic drainage, reducing the risk of complications such as seromas (fluid collections) and enhancing overall surgical outcomes. However, it is crucial to wear the faja as prescribed by your surgeon or healthcare provider, as excessive or improper use may lead to discomfort or complications.

Fajas are available in various sizes, and it is essential to find the right fit to ensure effective compression and support while maintaining comfort. Your surgeon or healthcare provider can guide you in selecting the appropriate faja based on your specific surgical procedure and individual needs. Following their recommendations and properly caring for the garment will contribute to a smoother and more successful recovery after surgery.

Note:

Indeed, the wide variety of compression garments or fajas available in the market can make it challenging to find the perfect fit based solely on descriptions or recommendations. Each person's body shape and surgical needs are unique, so what works well for one individual may not be the best choice for another.

The most reliable way to find the right faja for you is to discuss it with your surgeon or healthcare provider. They have a comprehensive understanding of your specific surgical procedure, the areas that require compression, and the level of support needed for optimal recovery. Your surgeon can recommend the appropriate type of faja that aligns with your postoperative needs and ensures proper compression in the targeted areas.

As your body heals and the swelling reduces during the recovery process, your size and shape may change. Therefore, it is essential to continuously assess the fit and comfort of your faja throughout the recovery period. Your surgeon may recommend adjustments or even changing to a different faja if necessary to accommodate the changes in your body and provide the best possible support.

When trying on or purchasing a faja, pay close attention to how it fits, ensuring that it provides adequate compression without being too tight or uncomfortable. Comfort is vital during the recovery period, so finding a faja that you can comfortably wear for extended periods is crucial to adherence and overall satisfaction with the garment.

In some cases, you may also be prescribed multiple fajas for different stages of your recovery. For example, you may start with a softer and more flexible garment immediately after surgery and then transition to a firmer, more supportive faja as your healing progresses.

Remember that the primary purpose of the faja is to support your recovery and promote proper healing after surgery. Following your surgeon's recommendations and staying in communication with them about your faja's fit and comfort will ensure you have the most effective and comfortable postoperative experience.

Tip:

Some LM therapists may offer faja alteration services in their offices, which can be incredibly beneficial for achieving a perfect fit and optimal compression. Fajas are designed to provide targeted support to specific areas of the body, and having a customized fit ensures that the compression is applied precisely where it is needed most.

When you opt for faja alteration services, the LM specialist will carefully assess your body's unique contours and surgical areas, making necessary adjustments to the garment. This can involve resizing the faja to ensure it conforms snugly to your body without being too tight or uncomfortable. Additionally, the therapist may modify the faja's length or other aspects to align with your body's dimensions and your specific recovery needs.

Having a faja that fits properly not only enhances its effectiveness in supporting your recovery but also enhances your overall comfort during the healing process. A well-fitted faja can help reduce swelling, minimize bruising, and improve the contour of the treated areas. Moreover, a properly adjusted faja can alleviate any discomfort or irritation that might arise from wearing an ill-fitting garment.

When discussing faja alteration options with your LM specialist, be sure to inquire about any additional costs or fees associated with the service. Also, ask about the timeframe for the alterations, as it may take some time to complete the adjustments to ensure precision and accuracy. The LM therapist will work closely with you to ensure your faja fits comfortably and supports your postoperative healing process effectively.

It's important to remember that faja alteration services provided by LM therapists are not meant to replace the guidance or recommendations of your surgeon. Always consult with your surgeon or healthcare provider before making any significant changes to your postoperative garments. By working collaboratively with your LM therapist and surgeon, you can optimize your recovery and achieve the best possible results after cosmetic surgery.

105

WHAT DO STAGES OF FAJAS MEAN?

One of the quintessential components of this recovery journey is the use of compression garments, popularly known as "fajas" in some cultures. Understanding the different stages of these garments can significantly influence the final results. Let's delve into the distinct stages of fajas and their specific purposes.

Stage 1: Immediate Post-Operative Faja

Duration: Typically worn for the first one to three weeks post-surgery.

Features:

- Made of high-compression fabric.
- Often features hooks, zippers, or both, for ease of use since mobility can be restricted right after surgery.
- Provides full coverage, often extending from the chest to the knees or ankles.

Purpose:

- Reduce Swelling: The immediate compression helps reduce post-operative edema.

- Support Healing: By holding everything in place, the faja can prevent complications like seromas or hematomas.
- Skin Adhesion: This initial compression aids the skin in adhering back to the underlying structures, essential for smooth results.

Stage 2: Intermediate Recovery Faja

Duration: Typically worn from the third week to the sixth or eighth week, depending on the surgeon's advice and individual healing.

Features:

- Gradually less restrictive than the stage one garment.
- Might have fewer hooks or zippers, and the fabric may be slightly softer.
- Offers a more contoured fit, aligning closely with the body's evolving shape.

Purpose:

- Continued Support: As the body heals and the initial swelling subsides, this faja continues to provide necessary support.
- Enhanced Mobility: Designed to be more flexible, allowing patients to return to daily activities with more ease.
- Shaping: As the body begins to adapt post-liposuction, this faja assists in refining the silhouette and ensuring even compression.

Stage 3: Final or Maintenance Faja

Duration: Can be worn after the eighth week and onwards, for several months or as advised by the surgeon.

Features:

- Made of breathable, flexible materials.

- Might resemble regular shapewear but still offers targeted compression.
- Easier to put on and often indistinguishable under clothing.

Purpose:

- Long-term Shaping: Helps in maintaining the liposuction results and ensuring the body contour remains as desired.
- Comfort: As the primary healing concludes, this faja provides support without causing discomfort, making it suitable for extended wear.
- Confidence Boost: Offers a sleeker appearance under clothing, boosting confidence as one showcases their new shape.

Note:

The transition from Stage 1 to Stage 2 faja usually occurs when the surgeon determines that the swelling has significantly reduced, and the body is healing well. The exact timing may vary from patient to patient, and it is essential to follow the surgeon's specific instructions regarding when to switch to Stage 2 faja.

Tip:

Selecting the correct faja (compression garment) after surgery is essential for optimal healing and comfort. Here are some tips to help you choose the right faja:

1. Consult with your surgeon: Always discuss the type of faja you need with your surgeon. They will provide specific recommendations based on the type of surgery you had, your body shape, and the areas that require compression.

2. Size and fit: Proper sizing is crucial for the effectiveness of the faja. It should fit snugly but not be too tight or

uncomfortable. Avoid choosing a faja that is too small, as it can cause discomfort and hinder circulation. A properly fitted faja will provide the right amount of compression to support your healing process.

3. Compression level: Consider the compression level required for your stage of recovery. Stage 1 fajas provide maximum compression for immediate postoperative recovery, while Stage 2 fajas offer a more moderate level of compression for the later stages of healing.

4. Material and construction: Look for fajas made from high-quality, breathable, and hypoallergenic materials that are gentle on the skin. Seamless and tag less designs can reduce irritation and discomfort.

5. Design and coverage: Ensure that the faja covers the treated areas adequately and offers support to the targeted regions. Some fajas may have specific designs for certain procedures (e.g., abdominal, buttocks, thighs), so choose one that aligns with your type of surgery.

6. Closure system: Consider the closure system of the faja, such as hooks, zippers, or adjustable straps. A closure system that allows for easy wear and removal will be more convenient during your recovery.

7. Comfort: This is essential during the healing process. Choose a faja that feels comfortable on your skin and doesn't cause excessive itching or irritation.

8. Durability: A high-quality faja should be durable and able to withstand regular wear and washing without losing its compression and shape.

9. Consult with an LM therapist: If possible, seek advice from a qualified LM therapist who has experience with

postoperative compression garments. They can help you select the right faja based on your specific needs and provide guidance on proper fitting and usage.

10. Purchase from a reputable source: Buy your faja from reputable retailers or medical supply stores to ensure the authenticity and quality of the product.

LEARN MORE:

Scan or click here to find out more about stages of fajas after surgery.

106

WHAT IS LIPO FOAM?

Lipo foam, also known as liposuction foam or compression foam, is a specialized medical device used in the postoperative care of patients who have undergone liposuction procedures or other surgical treatments. It is made from soft, pliable foam material and is designed to provide gentle and even pressure over the treated areas.

The primary purpose of lipo foam is to help distribute compression evenly and reduce the risk of irregularities or lumps forming in the skin after liposuction. By applying consistent pressure to the treated areas, lipo foam helps to prevent the accumulation of fluids, reduce swelling, and support the body's natural healing process.

Lipo foam is typically placed over the treated areas, secured with a compression garment or wrap, and worn for a certain period as advised by the surgeon or healthcare provider. It is often used in combination with compression garments to provide additional support and promote optimal results.

This medical device is generally well-tolerated and safe to use, but it is essential to follow the specific instructions provided by the surgeon or healthcare professional to ensure proper usage and avoid any potential complications.

Note:

In many cases, lipo foam is provided by the surgeon or obtained from the LM therapist, along with specific instructions on how to apply it correctly. Some LM offices even offer evaluation and adjustment (trimming) of lipo foam in the office, ensuring that it fits the patient's body shape perfectly and provides optimal compression and support.

It is important to note that while lipo foam is a valuable tool, it should always be used in conjunction with a comprehensive postoperative care plan prescribed by the surgeon or healthcare provider. This plan may include other post-surgical garments, manual lymphatic drainage, and dietary recommendations to further enhance the recovery process.

Tip:

Ask your LM therapist about different ways to trim lipofoam to fit perfectly under faja.

LEARN MORE:

Scan or click here to learn basic techniques of lipofoam trimming for better fit under compression garment.

_107_

WHAT TYPES OF LIPO FOAM ARE THERE?

When it comes to lipo foam, there are various options available on the market, each with slightly different textures and characteristics. Here is a comprehensive list of the available options:

1. **Standard Lipo Foam:** This is the most common type of lipo foam and is widely used after liposuction and body contouring procedures. It is made of soft, flexible foam material that provides gentle compression and support to the treated areas.

2. **Memory Lipo Foam:** This type is designed to conform to the body's contours more effectively. It molds to the specific shape of the body and retains that shape, providing a customized fit and enhanced comfort during the healing process.

3. **Adhesive Lipo Foam:** This type of lipo foam has an adhesive backing, allowing it to be easily secured to the skin or undergarments. The adhesive feature ensures that the foam

stays in place, even during movement, providing continuous compression and support.

4. **Silicone-Coated Lipo Foam:** This foam is designed to be non-stick and gentle on the skin. The silicone coating prevents the foam from adhering to wounds or incision sites, reducing the risk of irritation and discomfort.

5. **Perforated Lipo Foam:** This foam is characterized by small holes or perforations throughout the material. These perforations allow for improved breathability and ventilation, reducing the risk of moisture buildup and promoting better wound healing.

6. **Pre-Cut Lipo Foam:** Some lipo foam options come pre-cut into specific shapes and sizes, making them easy to apply and eliminating the need for trimming. These pre-cut pieces are often designed to fit common treatment areas, such as the abdomen, flanks, or thighs.

7. **Sterile Lipo Foam:** For patients with sensitive or delicate skin, sterile lipo foam is an ideal option. It is free of any potential irritants or contaminants, making it suitable for those with skin sensitivities.

Note:

When selecting the right lipo foam for postoperative care, it is essential to consult with the surgeon or LM therapist. They can recommend the most appropriate type based on the specific procedure performed, the patient's individual needs, and any postoperative concerns. Properly chosen lipo foam can significantly enhance the recovery process by providing the right amount of compression, support, and comfort for optimal healing and desired outcomes.

Tip:

When purchasing lipo foam online, it's essential to be mindful of the product's quality and pricing. While opting for the cheapest options may seem attractive due to their affordability, it's important to consider that the quality of these products might be compromised. Lipo foam that costs $13 or less may be made from lower-grade materials, which could result in reduced durability and effectiveness. Inferior quality foam may not provide adequate compression and support, potentially hindering the healing process and postoperative results.

On the other hand, the most expensive lipo foam options, priced over $25, may not necessarily offer significantly better quality compared to mid-priced alternatives. While some premium features may be included in these expensive products, they might not be necessary for all patients' needs. Paying a higher price for unnecessary features may not provide proportional benefits in terms of postoperative care and recovery.

Instead, it is often advisable to consider mid-priced lipo foam options, typically priced between $14 and $19. These products usually strike a good balance between affordability and quality. They are designed to provide the necessary compression and support, promoting optimal recovery without breaking the bank. Many mid-priced lipo foam options offer appropriate thickness and flexibility, ensuring effective use for various body contouring procedures.

Before making a purchase, it's beneficial to read customer reviews and product descriptions to gain insights into the foam's performance and suitability for postoperative use. Additionally, consulting with your surgeon or LM therapist can be helpful in selecting the most appropriate lipo foam based on individual needs and the specific surgical procedure performed.

LEARN MORE:

Scan or click <u>here</u> for tips on using Lipo Foam after plastic surgery.

108

HOW TO PLACE LIPO FOAM UNDER A FAJA AFTER 360 LIPO?

Put on a soft T-shirt or tank top first. Put on compression garment or faja over and bottom or hook halfway up. Place lipo foam pad sideways between faja and T-shirt on each side first. Push down until foam covers areas of liposuction. Place another piece of lipo foam over front of stomach in the same fashion. Adjust to avoid gaps or significant bulging due to overlap of sheets.

Note:

This is just a general example of lipo foam application and the exact application of lipo foam may vary in each individual case. Although initially this process is fairly cumbersome and may be sometimes uncomfortable, over time it becomes much easier.

Tip:

Multiple types of compression garments or fajas are available. Always follow the recommendation of your surgeon. However, among various types of fajas, most patients find compression garments with an opening in the perineal area (aka "peehole") most useful since those do not require re-application of the foam after each time you use the bathroom.

LEARN MORE:

Scan or click here to learn tips for cleaning postoperative garments.

109

HOW MANY LIPO FOAM PADS DO I NEED FOR COMPRESSION AFTER BODY SURGERY SUCH AS ABDOMINOPLASTY OR 360 LIPOSUCTION?

The number of lipo foam pads needed for compression after 360 liposuction can vary depending on the individual, the specific surgical areas treated, and the surgeon's recommendations. Typically, patients will require multiple lipo foam pads to cover the entire treated area adequately.

For 360 liposuction, which involves liposuction of the abdomen, waist, and thighs, you may need at least four to six lipo foam pads. This would allow you to cover the entire treated area and ensure uniform compression, which is crucial for effective postoperative care.

To determine the exact number of lipo foam pads you need, it's essential to consult with your surgeon or LM therapist. They can assess your specific situation, the extent of the liposuction, and any other factors that may influence the postoperative care requirements.

During your follow-up appointments after the procedure, your healthcare professional can also evaluate how well the lipo foam is working for you and make any necessary adjustments or additions to ensure optimal results and a smooth recovery process.

Note:

It is highly likely that more than one set of lipo foam pads will be required throughout the recovery process. In the early stages of recovery, there may be some leakage of body fluids through the incisions and drain sites, which can potentially stain the lipo foam. While lipo foam can be washed and reused multiple times, each time it may lose some of its softness and texture. Over time, lipo foam may also gradually become discolored due to oxidation, taking on a yellowish appearance. Although discolored lipo foam is still functional, many individuals prefer to use new ones due to the unsightly appearance.

To ensure effective compression and comfort during the recovery period, it is essential to have an adequate supply of lipo foam on hand. As lipo foam may need to be changed or washed regularly, having more than one set allows you to maintain a clean and hygienic compression garment.

Discussing the use of lipo foam with your surgeon or LM therapist can be helpful, as they can provide specific guidance on how many sets of lipo foam you may need and how to care for them properly. By following their recommendations and ensuring a sufficient supply, you can promote a smooth and successful recovery after 360 liposuction.

Tip:

When it comes to selecting the right lipo foam pads for your postoperative recovery, it can be beneficial to explore various options to find the one that suits you best. Many manufacturers offer sample packs containing lipo foam pads from different brands, which allows you to try out different types and assess their comfort, fit, and performance.

By purchasing sample packs, you can test how each lipo foam pad feels against your skin, how well it conforms to your body's contours, and whether it provides adequate compression and support. This can be particularly helpful as individual preferences and sensitivities can vary, and what works well for one person may not be as suitable for another.

Consider trying lipo foam pads from two to three different manufacturers to compare their quality and features. Look for options with varying textures, thicknesses, and sizes to see which one feels the most comfortable and supportive for you. Pay attention to factors such as breathability, ease of washing and maintenance, and whether they cause any skin irritation.

Additionally, during the recovery period, your body's needs may change, and what feels comfortable initially might not be the best choice later on. Having a variety of lipo foam pads to choose from can be advantageous as you can switch to a different one if needed.

Ultimately, selecting the right lipo foam pads will enhance your overall postoperative experience and promote a smoother recovery. Take the time to try out different options and consult with your surgeon or LM therapist for their recommendations to find the lipo foam pads that best meet your needs and preferences.

LEARN MORE:

Scan or click <u>here</u> to learn about different types of postoperative compression foam pads.

110

WHAT IS AN ABDOMINAL BOARD?

An abdominal board is a compression garment accessory commonly used after abdominal plastic surgery, liposuction, or tummy tuck procedures. It is a flat, firm, and rigid board typically made of foam or other durable materials. The board is designed to be placed on the abdomen underneath the compression garment or faja to provide additional support and compression to the treated area.

The main purpose of the abdominal board is to help distribute pressure evenly across the abdominal region, reducing the risk of fluid buildup (seroma) and promoting more even healing and contouring of the treated area. By providing extra compression, it also helps to minimize swelling and assists in shaping the waistline and abdominal muscles.

Abdominal boards come in different sizes to accommodate various body shapes and surgical needs. Some boards have adjustable straps or fasteners to secure them in place under the compression garment, while others are simply placed inside the garment.

It is essential to follow your surgeon's or LM therapist's recommendations regarding the proper use of the abdominal board after surgery. They will guide you on how long to wear it, how to position it correctly, and when it can be removed during your recovery process. Proper and consistent use of the abdominal board can contribute to better results and a smoother recovery after abdominal procedures.

Note:

The abdominal board and lipo foam serve different purposes during the recovery process after abdominal surgery or liposuction. While both are used to provide compression and support, the choice of when to use each depends on the stage of recovery and individual comfort.

During the initial phase of recovery, the abdomen can be more sensitive, swollen, and tender. This is when lipo foam is typically utilized as it offers a softer and more flexible compression. Lipo foam pads can be easily adjusted and contoured to fit the body's curves, providing a gentler and more accommodating compression over the treated areas. This helps to reduce the risk of excessive pressure on the still healing tissues and makes it more comfortable for the patient.

As the recovery progresses and the abdomen becomes less sensitive, patients may start to tolerate firmer compression. This is when the abdominal board comes into play. The board offers a more rigid and uniform compression, which can be beneficial for achieving optimal contouring and reducing swelling. However, because of its firmer nature, it may cause some discomfort if applied too early in the recovery process.

The transition from lipo foam to the abdominal board typically occurs around one to four weeks post-surgery, depending on the individual's healing progress and the surgeon's recommendations. It's crucial to follow the guidance of your healthcare provider or LM therapist when deciding on the appropriate time to switch to the abdominal board.

Remember that both lipo foam and the abdominal board are meant to enhance the healing process and provide support during the recovery journey. Following the recommended timeline and guidelines for their use can help ensure a more comfortable and successful recovery after abdominal surgery or liposuction.

Tip:

When considering the use of an abdominal compression board, it's essential to be aware that these boards come in various shapes and sizes to accommodate different body types and surgical procedures. Consulting with your surgeon or LM therapist can provide valuable insights and recommendations on selecting the most suitable abdominal board for your specific needs.

During your postoperative recovery, your healthcare provider or LM therapist will assess your healing progress and individual anatomy to determine the appropriate abdominal board for you. They may consider factors such as the extent of your surgical procedure, the location and size of incisions, and the level of swelling and bruising in the abdominal area.

Some abdominal boards are designed to be more flexible, allowing for contouring to the body's curves, while others may have a more rigid construction for a uniform and consistent compression. Your surgeon or LM therapist will take these factors into account and suggest the best option to support your recovery.

Additionally, they can provide guidance on how to properly use the abdominal board for optimal results. They may advise you on the duration of use, how to secure the board in place, and any adjustments needed to ensure comfort and effectiveness.

LEARN MORE:

Scan or click <u>here</u> to learn more about benefits of using an abdominal board.

GLOSSARY:

Lymphatic Massage (LM): A therapy focusing on stimulating the lymphatic system to improve fluid removal from the body, especially useful after surgery to reduce swelling and aid healing.

Manual Lymphatic Drainage (MLD): Techniques used in LM involving specific, repetitive strokes to move fluid from swollen areas into the lymphatic vessels and nodes.

Edema Fluid: Excess fluid accumulated in body tissues, often causing swelling. LM mobilizes this fluid into the lymphatic system.

Lymphatic System: A network of tissues and organs in the body that helps rid the body of toxins and waste. It transports lymph, a fluid containing infection-fighting white blood cells.

Detoxification: The process of removing toxins, excess fluids, and waste from the body. LM aids this process by stimulating the lymphatic system.

Fibrosis: The thickening and scarring of connective tissue, usually as a result of injury. LM may be needed to address persistent edema or fibrosis.

Superficial Lymph Vessels: Tiny vessels located just under the skin. LM targets these vessels to move stagnant fluid from swollen areas back into the lymphatic system.

Lymph Nodes: Small structures that filter lymph fluid. LM typically starts at major lymph nodes to improve overall lymph flow.

Cavitation: A technique used in body contouring, involving the use of ultrasound waves to break down fat cells.

Seroma: A condition where fluid accumulates in a region of the body, often occurring after surgery.

Hematoma: A solid swelling of clotted blood within the tissues.

Kinesiology Tape: A type of elastic therapeutic tape used for treating athletic injuries and a variety of physical disorders.

Wood Therapy: A technique using wooden instruments to massage and sculpt the body, often used in postoperative care to aid in the healing process.

Arnica Montana: An herb used in homeopathic medicine to reduce swelling and bruising.

Bromelain: An enzyme found in pineapples, known for its anti-inflammatory properties, often used to reduce swelling.

Curcumin: The active compound in turmeric, renowned for its potent anti-inflammatory properties.

Faja: A Spanish term for a compression garment used after body contouring procedures to aid in recovery.

Lipo Foam: Foam pads used under compression garments after liposuction to ensure even pressure on the treated areas.

Abdominal Board: A board placed under compression garments to provide even pressure and support in the abdominal area after surgery.

BBL (Brazilian Butt Lift): A cosmetic procedure involving the transfer of fat to enhance the size and shape of the buttocks.

CoolSculpting: A non-surgical body contouring procedure that freezes and eliminates fat cells.

AFTERWORD:

Thank you for taking the time to read our book. We have endeavored to present the material in a clear and accessible manner, aiming to enhance your understanding of lymphatic massage following plastic surgery. It's important to emphasize that the information provided here is educational and not a substitute for professional medical advice. This book is designed to facilitate informed discussions with your surgeon and lymphatic massage specialist, aiding you in making well-informed and safe decisions about your postoperative care.

We strongly advise using sound judgment and consulting with a healthcare professional before attempting any techniques or using products mentioned in this book. Your safety and a swift recovery are our utmost priorities. If you found this book helpful, we would be grateful if you could share it with others who might benefit from it as well. Additionally, leaving a review on Amazon would greatly help in making this resource more accessible to a broader audience. For any suggestions or further information, please feel free to visit the authors' page. We wish you a smooth and safe recovery journey.

Max Yeslev, MD, Ruth Mueller, LMT

Made in the USA
Columbia, SC
28 October 2024

44822737R00189